D0096435

NOW

I

KIDS
TELL KIDS
ABOUT
SAFETY

KNOW

BETTER,
too

Yale New Haven Health

NOW I KNOW BETTER, *too*

KIDS TELL KIDS ABOUT SAFETY

Copyright © 1999 by Yale New Haven Health
All rights reserved.

This book may not be reproduced, in whole or in part, including illustrations,
in any form (beyond that copying permitted by Sections 107 and 108 of the
U.S. Copyright Law and except by reviewers for the public press),
without written permission from the publisher.

To the children of Connecticut

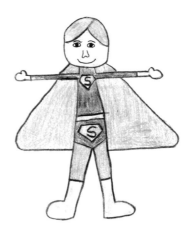

Contents

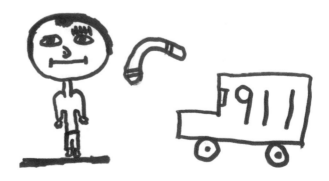

Note from Governor Rowland

 As governor of Connecticut, I am proud to represent a state that is committed to the health and safety of its children. First, let me share the following facts. After age 1, more children are killed by injuries than by all diseases combined. The leading cause of injury and death is motor vehicle accidents. For ages 1-4, the next leading causes of accidental deaths are fires/burns, drowning, suffocation, and firearms. For ages 5-14, the leading causes of accidental deaths, after motor vehicles, are firearms, drowning, fires/burns, and suffocation.

These statistics are alarming, but issues that affect the people of Connecticut, especially our children, should not be viewed in terms of just statistics. So let me speak to you as a parent.

There can be no greater tragedy than to have a child die or become disabled because of an accident that might have been prevented. This is what *Now I Know Better, Too* is all about. The first edition, published in 1996, was a success throughout Connecticut—in fact, it was read and written about from Los Angeles to Boston, from Chicago to Miami. As parents, we know that our kids often listen more to other kids than to adults. This is why these stories have reached children all around the country.

We in Connecticut have made a strong investment in preventive health care. For example, the HUSKY program, Healthcare for Uninsured Kids and Youth, serves children up to age 19 with a comprehensive package of benefits ranging from preventive care to eyeglasses. It makes so much more sense to prevent illness or accidents from happening in the first place, than to have to deal with the pain, the trauma, and the financial burdens afterward.

Connecticut has shown the foresight to enact legislation and support cooperative efforts to improve the health and the lives of our citizens, especially those who cannot necessarily speak for themselves. On the other hand, we should not underestimate the abilities of our children. As you will see in *Now I Know Better, Too,* they speak pretty well for themselves, in powerful, personal messages that will reach others.

I congratulate Yale New Haven Health on this public-service endeavor. Connecticut's legislators, parents, schools, and health-care providers share many common bonds. Our mutual goal is the best health possible for all of our children.

John G. Rowland
Governor, State of Connecticut

Note from the Editors

When the first edition of *Now I Know Better* was published in 1996, the idea that kids would listen to other kids talking about preventing injuries sounded like it might work. As adults, we already knew that kids often pay more attention to other kids than they do to grown-ups.

What we didn't realize was how successful *Now I Know Better* would become. The stories told by the children of Connecticut in their own words rang true with every child who picked up the book. Almost universally, parents reported that when their youngsters started to read the book, the children kept reading until they finished all the stories. This is a tribute to the 70 children whose stories and advice on safety and accident prevention were included in the 1996 book.

Subsequently, a half-hour video edition of *Now I Know Better* was broadcast on Connecticut Public Television and distributed throughout the state. Guida Milk and Ice Cream Company collaborated with NBC 30-WVIT and Yale-New Haven Children's Hospital to print children's safety messages on more than 1 million milk cartons used in schools and sold in stores.

In the fall of 1998, Yale New Haven Health again turned to children to ask for stories written in their own words about how other kids could remain safe and avoid injuries. Once again, Connecticut's children responded enthusiastically with more than 1,200 stories, nearly double the number submitted for the first book.

We would like to extend our thanks to the parents and teachers who encouraged their children and students to tell their stories. We also would like to thank our colleagues in the Emergency Department who helped to select the stories included in this volume.

Most important, we thank the children of Connecticut who offered their good advice so that others won't be hurt.

Douglas Baker, M.D.   Thomas Kennedy, M.D.
Yale-New Haven Children's Hospital   *Bridgeport Hospital*

Kevin Smothers, M.D.
Greenwich Hospital

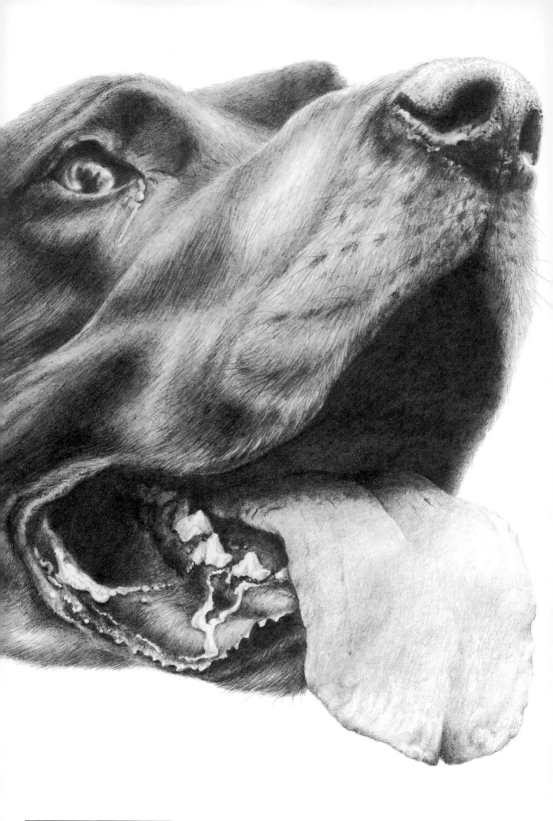

Asthma

A Dangerous Visit

One night, I wanted to sleep over my friend Jay's house. My parents did not think it was a good idea. I am allergic to dogs, and Jay has a Black Lab. That night, I struggled to breathe. The next morning, breathing became more and more difficult.

About 7:30 in the morning, Jay's mom brought me home, my mom called 911, and an ambulance arrived at about 8:00. I was having a severe asthma attack. My mom told me later that I was drooling and almost unconscious. I was put on so many medications I was shaking. The doctors in the emergency room also gave me an inhaler that had a long tube on the end. I didn't have anything to eat that morning, so my mom got me a doughnut from the hospital's vending machine. I was at the hospital almost all day.

My advice to people with asthma and allergies: Please be wise. While visiting homes where people have pets, use medicine before entering.

Ryan Bonomo, 13
Vernon

Dr. Baker's Comment:
Children who have asthma often also have allergies. Their asthma will sometimes be less severe if they avoid contact with whatever they are allergic to. If Ryan had taken his parent's advice, he could have prevented a trip to the hospital.

When parents suggest something that you don't agree with, there is often a good reason.

It's Worth the Trouble!

I have chronic asthma and need many different types of inhalers and sprays to breathe. One night, I went to bed without taking my allergy and asthma medications. What a mistake! I was half-asleep when I realized that I had forgotten to take them, but I thought I should just get a good night's sleep instead.

The next morning, when I woke up, my mom asked me how I felt. My eyes were bloodshot, and I had developed a whooping cough—a loud hacking cough that hurts. I tried to put in my soft contacts. Rejected! I tried to breathe for a minute without a single cough. Couldn't! I stayed home from school with a sinus headache and a sickening cough that day, all because I was too lazy to take my medicine.

All kids reading this: Remember to take your medicine!

Tucker George, 13
West Hartford

Dr. Baker's Comment:

One of the most common reasons why medicines do not work is because people forget to take them. Remember, it is important to take your medicine. If you don't, you'll just become ill, when you could have stayed well instead.

Axes

Bloody Toes

While my mom, my brother, and I were visiting some friends, my five-year-old brother, Kyle, went outside to play. He found an axe by a wood pile and picked it up, but it slipped out of his hands and landed on his toe. He screamed a blood-curdling scream. My mother heard him and ran outside to see what was wrong. Kyle was sitting on the ground holding his ankle, and his sneakers were soaked with blood. My mom picked him up and carried him into the house. She gently took off his sneaker, not knowing what to expect. He was bleeding a lot. She was afraid that he had cut off one of his toes. Mom's friend called the doctor, who had an office not far from her house. My mom carried Kyle to the car, and we all piled in. The doctor cut Kyle's sock off. He had a cut and a huge blood blister under his toenail. To relieve the pressure, the doctor stuck a needle into Kyle's toenail. Kyle was really in a lot of pain. He couldn't wear shoes for a while, and his foot bothered him for a couple of weeks.

The lesson I learned from this experience is never to touch or play with things that belong to someone else. Also, always ask the permission of an adult before you pick up any type of tools or dangerous equipment.

Brittany Hallenbeck, 13
Burlington

Dr. Smothers's Comment:

Boy, have I heard a lot of stories like this one! Too many children have access to sharp, dangerous tools—whether they are axes, knives, or power tools. Just ask Brittany and Kyle.

Kids need to pay close attention to what they pick up to play with and should only handle tools when they have an adult's permission. Parents should also spend time with their children, working on a project, to show them how to handle tools properly—and to have some fun at the same time.

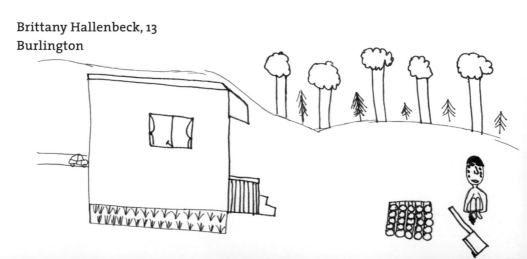

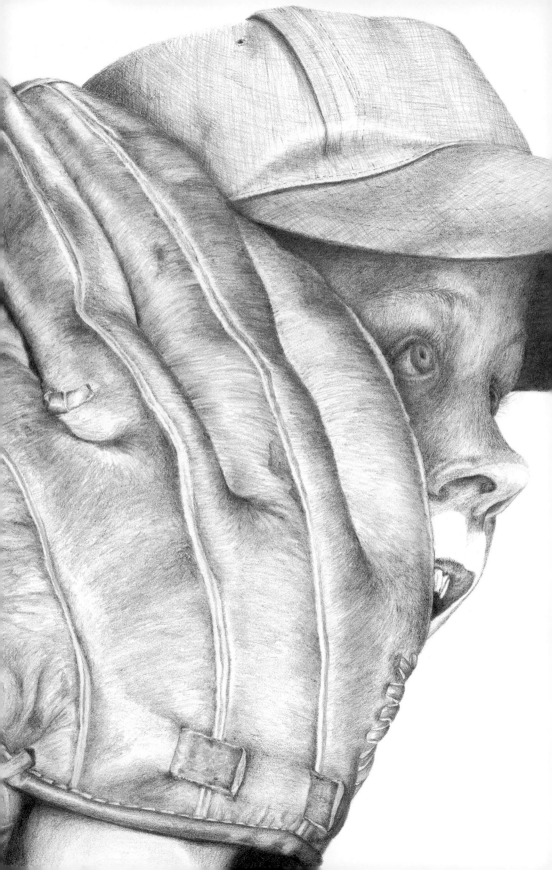

Baseball

Catch!

Raising my worn leather glove, I crouched down to catch the baseball my brother was about to whip toward me. I caught his warm-up pitches with ease, and gradually began to lose interest in the game. Suddenly, Spencer threw the ball aggressively. I turned sideways and blocked my face with the mitt. The ball struck the side of my mouth, and I felt the impact through the glove. Clutching my face, I felt bits of tooth floating around in my saliva. I spit them out in disgust and hollered, "Mom!" I saw horror on her face as I showed her what happened.

She phoned my orthodontist, Dr. Drew, who requested an immediate examination. Nancy, my favorite orthodontic assistant, led me to the dentist's chair, which was fully equipped with strange gadgets. Dr. Drew said, "Open your mouth and let me see." I opened wide. A sigh of relief came from him as he explained, "The ball did do some damage, but your tooth will heal nicely."

When playing a sport, always focus on the game—or stop playing. Most sports move swiftly and involve flying objects. If your mind is on something else when you step onto the playing field, you may not be as fortunate as I was and could become seriously injured.

Andrew Glantz, 12
West Hartford

Dr. Smothers's Comment:
Ouch! Who said baseball was not a contact sport?

Whether you are a player or a spectator, you should always be alert when it comes to sports. Play it safe. Wear protective equipment, such as helmets, face guards, and shin guards. Play on safe, level fields, free of glass and other debris. And always pay attention to what is going on around you!

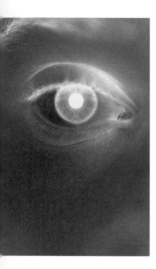

The Hunchback of Notre Dame

Two years ago, I was first-base coaching when the coach called me over to the dugout. Without thinking, I removed my helmet and started to trot over to him, past home plate. Out of the corner of my eye, I noticed the kid on deck's bat quickly approaching my head. His bat connected with my face. I never really blacked out, but what happened next is pretty foggy. I remember someone bringing a snow cone over to put on my gash, and I thought they were going to let me eat it. My dad brought me to the hospital, where people took X rays.

By the time I got home, my eye was swollen shut. I looked like the Hunchback of Notre Dame. On my first day back in school, my whole left eye was totally red. The doctor said that blood had gotten caught in part of my eye.

This accident could have been completely avoided if I had not been so ignorant. I know that helmets in sports are uncomfortable and look funny, but I look better in a helmet than I do as the Hunchback.

Greg Hom, 13
Harwinton

Keep Your Eye on that Ball!

One night, I went with my dad, cousin, and friend to see the New York Mets play the visiting Arizona Diamondbacks. We sat near first base, and I brought my glove with me. After the fourth inning, the announcer said that we could move to closer seats because there were not a lot of people there that night. It was the top of the fifth inning, and as we were moving, a Diamondback batter hit a foul ball that popped up. It was a pretty cool sight! It was at least a few feet away from me, and I thought it would not hit me so I took my eye off the ball. When I looked again, the ball had curved very fast. I should have caught it, but instead the ball hit me on my mouth. I suddenly realized that I was bleeding and one of my teeth had fallen out.

I was immediately taken to see the doctor. (On the way to get checked out, I saw Andy Benes, a pitcher for the Diamondbacks!) I was given ice for the swelling and was very frightened. The impact of the ball chipped my front tooth, and two of my teeth came out. Of course, when we went home, my mom was very surprised to see my face. She said that of all people in the baseball park, you were the lucky one that got hit! In my seven years of playing softball, I was never hit like that. Now I know to always keep my eyes on the ball and pay attention.

Nathan Rivera, 13
Stamford

Bicycles

Helmets Help

My name is Isaac. I am eight years old. This is my story.

I was riding my bike on a beautiful summer day. I was going down a hill and lost control. I hit a pothole and flew over the bike into the air about 10 feet away. I landed on my head, face first! Lucky for me, I was wearing a helmet. I think if I hadn't been wearing one, my head would have cracked. The helmet showed how bad my accident was. A chunk of the helmet was missing, and the paint came off. Below the helmet, my face was cut very badly. A neighbor who was a nurse saw what happened and waited with me for the ambulance. I spent many hours at the hospital.

My advice to any kids who ride bikes is to walk their bikes down steep hills, watch for potholes, and always wear a helmet. It saved my head and my brain and possibly my life.

Isaac Civitello, 8
Waterbury

Dr. Baker's Comment:

No matter how careful you are, accidents can still happen. Luckily, Isaac was wearing a safety helmet, which is what all bike riders should do. I have no doubt that, by wearing his helmet, Isaac avoided a much more serious injury. Well done, Isaac!

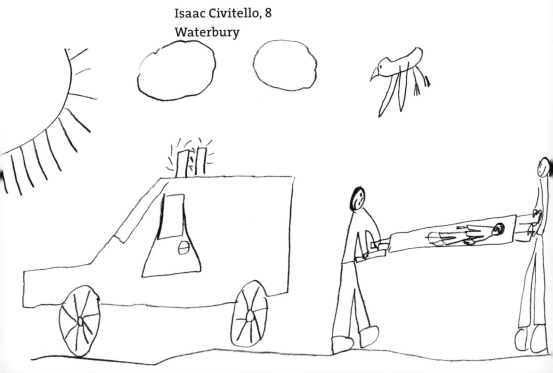

Lucky...This Time

When I was ten, I asked my Mom if I could go bike riding. I remember her saying, "Well, okay, but be careful because there is sand on the road." I decided I would go up the big hill in front of my house and ride down so that I could go really fast—but that was a mistake I would regret! I was at the top of the hill, all out of breath. My friend Ashley and her mother were walking by at the time. "Okay, here I go!" I said. I sped down the hill so fast I lost control. I remember sliding and falling face first on the ground. The pain killed. I felt as if I had been shot with 100 needles at the same time.

Dr. Baker's Comment:
Because she was wearing her helmet, Deena was only cut badly when she fell from her bike. Many children are injured more seriously. Helmets save lives! Be sure you are wearing yours whenever you ride your bike.

Ashley's mother ran to get me and brought me to my mother. It was horrible. Everyone was crying, especially me. They rushed me to the emergency room. The bike had fallen on my leg so my dad carried me. They put me on a long bed, and my mom held my hand tightly. After a while, I felt strings pulling on my chin. I was getting stitches. The doctor said, "Deena, it was a good thing you were wearing your helmet, but next time ride with caution. If this happens again, your chin might not be fixable."

I don't want what happened to me to happen to you. Always wear your helmet and ride cautiously because next time—well, there might not be a next time.

Deena Deragopian, 13
Stratford

Trust Your Instincts

One day, three of my friends and I were riding bikes. We got bored so we said, "Let's make a bike trail in the woods." We made a trail that started at the top of the steepest hill. First, we let my friend's bike go down with no one on it. The bike hit a rock and flipped. Then, another friend rode down on his bike with his brakes on. He tried it twice more without the brakes on and made it to the bottom.

Dr. Baker's Comment:

If your instincts are telling you that something is dangerous, it probably is. Trust your instincts—or ask an adult for safety advice to keep yourself and your friends out of dangerous situations. There are plenty of things to do that are both fun and safe.

After that, we went to my house to call more people, but when we got back to the trail it was almost dark. We told Chris to ride down, but I said, "No! It's almost dark. You can't see any stumps or rocks." Everyone agreed with me. Not following the group's advice, Chris went down anyway, hit a tree stump, flipped, and landed on the ground. Everyone screamed, "Are you okay?" He screamed, "I broke my arm, I broke my arm."

I ran to a nearby market to call 911. A police car drove by with the sirens on, so I waved it down. A lot of cars stopped to help. Then, I waved the ambulance down. The paramedics went down the trail to look at Chris. They said he had a compound fracture—that's when your bone sticks out of your skin. The paramedics put him in the ambulance and sped off to the hospital. They set his arm in a cast and said he would have a full recovery.

I am happy that I listened to my instincts, which told me that no one should have attempted that ride. My instincts also helped me act quickly to notify people.

Seeing someone have an accident is not fun. My friends and I learned that it is not smart to take chances

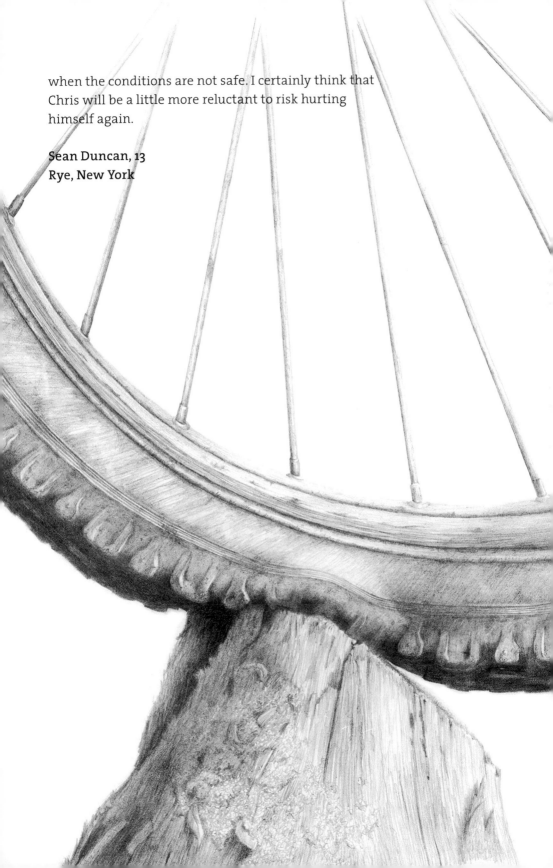

when the conditions are not safe. I certainly think that Chris will be a little more reluctant to risk hurting himself again.

Sean Duncan, 13
Rye, New York

Think First, Fly Later

One day, we went to our friends' house for dinner. It was a dark, gloomy-looking day. The sun was buried in clouds. It seemed like something bad was about to happen.

Dr. Baker's Comment:

Jason learned the hard way that safety comes first. Always be certain that you know how to ride someone else's bike before you try it. And, of course, always put on your safety gear before taking off.

Before dinner, we rode bikes. I hopped on my bike and dashed off because I was way behind the others. I didn't notice that I wasn't wearing my helmet. Also, I was riding a bike with hand brakes. At the time, I was used to coaster brakes. I had no clue that this might lead me to trouble later. I followed my friend into someone else's driveway. Everything happened fast. First, my mom ran out the door yelling at me, but I didn't understand her words. I cut across the lawn to get to the driveway. Next, I saw some stones ahead of me, so I peddled backward to stop. That didn't work, so I grabbed onto a shrub. That only flung me around backward and upside down. I landed on the driveway on my head, with the bicycle on top of me. It hurt—a lot! Afterward, all I remembered was being dizzy with blurry vision. Then I felt an ice pack against my head.

Three hours later, at the Yale-New Haven Children's Hospital, I found out that I had flown off a 3-foot-high stone wall. The doctors told me that I had a concussion. I can tell you right now that you should always wear a helmet and know how to drive your vehicle properly if you don't want to get hurt. A helmet might look funny, but a hospital cast looks worse!

Jason Hirth, 13
Orange

A Lesson I'll Never Forget

I've tried to forget it, but it won't go away. It was a crisp autumn day, late in the afternoon. My friend Max and I glided down the street on our shiny new bikes. We had lived in the same neighborhood for our whole lives and had been best friends for as long as I can remember. We loved cruising down the street on our bikes, going off homemade ramps. We walked our bikes to the top of the hill. We were going to race to the bottom, which meant going around a dangerous corner. "Go!" I shouted, and we were off. Max zoomed out ahead, not slowing down for the corner, when, suddenly, his wheels hit the sand in the road, unable to grip. He and the bike went skidding sideways and came to a crashing stop. To make things worse, a car zoomed around the corner at the same time, crashing into Max. I slammed on my brakes and dodged the car, veering off into the woods. I hit a root and flipped head over handlebars to the ground. Blood trickled down my face. "Max!" I thought. I limped over to the accident, and crouched down, not wanting to look under the car, but knowing I had to. There was Max, his little body in a deranged position. What had I done to my friend? I ran around screaming for help. George, a retired doctor, came running out of his house. George got Max out from under the car with the help of the driver and myself, but it was too late. Max was dead.

My advice to you is to be careful on your bike and always wear a helmet. Bikes can be fun, but should not cost you your life.

Hallie Macdonald, 13
Bristol

Bites

A Fuzzy Friend?

One day, I was walking with my best friend by our favorite little creek near our house. Sitting by the creek, I suddenly saw a tiny, fat, brown animal come creeping out of a hole. "Oh, look!" I cried. "That must be the little mole my dad was talking about!" Without thinking, I bent down to pet it. It had a soft, fuzzy coat and adorable paws—and sharp buck teeth! You can probably guess what happened next. He bit my finger and ran into another hole.

I stared at my finger. There was a small cut and a tiny drop of blood. "It doesn't look bad," my friend said. "C'mon, let's go for a walk." I was a little worried, but eventually I forgot about the mole's little nibble.

When I got home later, I said matter-of-factly to my parents, "Oh, by the way, that mole that you saw, he bit me!" Oops. Pandemonium! My parents both started yelling at once, and I got scared when they said I might have to get rabies shots. We didn't know whether moles carried rabies, but rabies make animals act strangely, and moles usually don't come out in the daylight. My mom made me scrub with soap and warm water for 15 minutes while she called the emergency room. She got off the phone and said, "You were lucky this time! Moles don't get rabies." I was so relieved, I almost fell off my chair.

Dr. Baker's Comment:

Exploring nature is fun, but sometimes it's also dangerous. A wild animal's first instinct is to defend itself against enemies. Maggie's friend the mole was just trying to stay safe. Remember to always give animals a safe zone. Staying outside that zone will help everyone enjoy the outdoors.

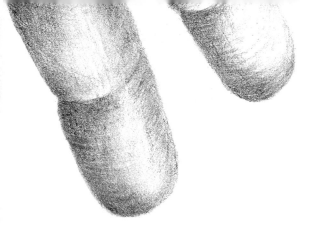

This accident shouldn't have happened, but it did, due to my foolishness. Don't make my mistake. Think before touching or petting wild animals or animals that you don't know.

Maggie Moore, 11
Trumbull

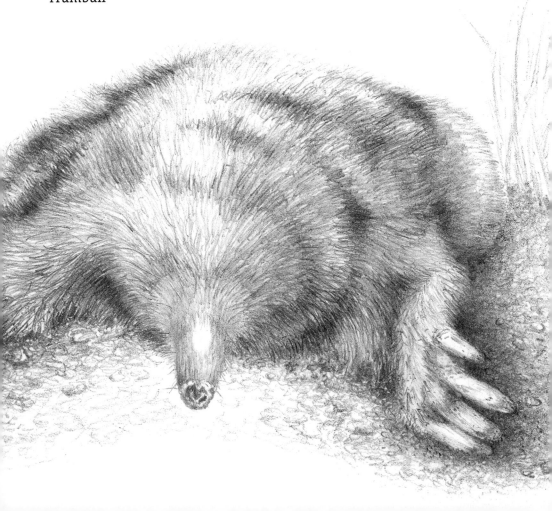

Boomerangs

Look Out!

Sean, my eight-year-old brother, was at a birthday party, and each guest received a plastic boomerang. The kids were in the backyard, throwing around their new toys. Sean bent down to pick up his boomerang, and when he stood up, he got hit in the head with the speeding boomerang that his friend had just thrown. It hit him about 2 inches above his left eyebrow.

Sean's friend's mom told my mom to wrap some ice in a piece of cloth and put it on the wound. My mom rushed Sean to the hospital. He received about five stitches. If you and a friend are playing with boomerangs, make sure that you both know where each other is before you throw. Keep an eye on the boomerang, too, so you know where it is at all times. Hopefully, you won't get hurt and have to go to the hospital like my brother.

Melissa Harrigan, 12
Harwinton

Dr. Smothers's Comment:
Who do parents still buy boomerangs as toys for children? There really is no safe way to play with those things. In the hands of children and inexperienced adults, accidents like Sean's will happen. My motto is, "Ban Boomerangs."

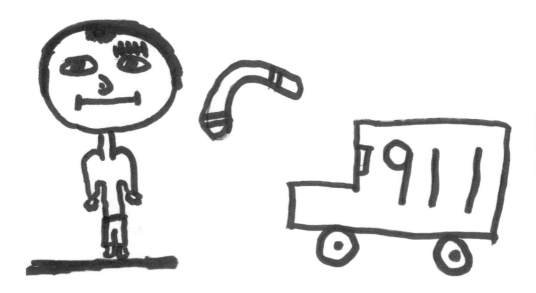

Burns

Tips for Cooks

One day, I was making breakfast for my mom. My dad was on a business trip. My mom was upstairs in her room. I put the eggs in the pan and put the pan on the stove. I turned on the burner and went to watch TV until I thought it was time to turn over the eggs.

Later, when I went to look at the eggs, they were not cooking, so I turned the burner higher to make the eggs cook faster. I thought that maybe I had turned on the wrong burner, so I touched the burner with my fingers to check. It was not hot. Then I touched the next burner, and it was not hot. I tried the next one. It was really, really hot! Before I could run cold water on my fingers to make them feel better, the skin started to blister.

I started bouncing around because my finger really hurt! Then I started to cry. My mom heard me and came downstairs to see what had happened. I told her everything, and she understood. I had to soak my three fingers in ice water for two hours. Then, I put an aloe vera ointment on them.

This experience taught me never to go near a stove without a parent nearby. It also taught me to tell my parents when something bad happens to me because they will understand and try to help.

Katharine Bischoff, 10
Southbury

Dr. Baker's Comment:
The kitchen can be a dangerous place. Although it is fun to help prepare meals, children should not try to cook unless they have an adult helping them. Burns, cuts, and other injuries can happen quickly and easily.

How to Handle Handles

When my sister was 11 months old, she rolled into the kitchen in her walker. My mom was making dinner. My sister rolled by the stove, reached up, and accidentally pulled down a pot of steaming hot water. It spilled all over her. For a long time after that, she had to wear bandages all over her body. Now she is 12 years old and has scars on her foot and arm and a bald spot on her head. Remember—and remind your parents—to always turn the handle of a pot or pan away from the edge of the stove.

Kimberly Nicole Catlin, 10
Bridgeport

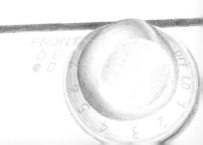

Fire and Water

My friend and I were cooking a meal for her mom on Mother's Day. We put out nice glasses, shiny silverware, and colorful plates. We wanted to make pasta first, but we had to get her mother out of the kitchen! We finally got her out of the kitchen and set a pot of water to boil on the stove. When the water boiled, we took the pot off the stove and put it on the counter, which we thought was stable (it was not). The pot fell, and water splashed everywhere, including all over us. My friend screamed, but I could only shiver in fright. Quickly, my friend's mom put ice on us and called my dad. He drove me to the hospital. They took off all the dead skin and then bandaged me up. Within the next month, my arm had only a scar, which is still there. Hot water is just as bad as a fire.

Rebecca Wortman, 10
New Haven

Dr. Baker's Comment:
Taking the time to be careful is well worth it, as Rebecca now knows. Cooking for your mother is a thoughtful thing to do, but other surprises can be just as nice—and much less hazardous.

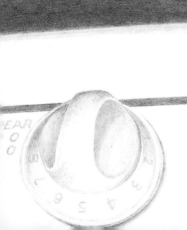

Learning the Hard Way

Easter Sunday, when I was four years old, my mother was getting my sister and I ready for our church's morning service. She was going to straighten our hair with a straightening comb (an iron comb that heats up on an ignited stove isle). She was about to press my hair when my sister told her that she could not find her slip. My mother turned off the isle and brought us both upstairs while she tried to find the slip. She was searching the closets when I decided to sneak downstairs to the kitchen. I hated getting my hair straightened and decided to do it myself.

Dr. Baker's Comment:
Children should never go near open flames. Jariba is very fortunate not to have been more seriously injured. Take her advice: Stay clear of fires, big and small.

Thinking that the fire itself would straighten my hair, I stuck the tips of my bangs into the flames. The next thing I knew my entire head was on fire, and I was screaming for my mother. She rushed downstairs and patted the flames out with her nightgown. She called an ambulance and then called my father to bring me to Bridgeport Hospital.

I returned home that night but had to go back to the hospital a few weeks later to receive an operation called a skin graft. The doctors took skin from my left thigh to cover the burn mark I had on my forehead. I remained in the hospital for about a week.

Several times before that accident, I had thought about asking my mother how fire straightened hair, but I never did. My advice is, if you have any questions concerning fire, ask. Fire is not a toy, and young children should keep their distance. I am just sorry that I had to learn the hard way.

Jariba Lynette Dawkins, 17
Stratford

Very, Very Hot Cocoa

It was about 8 p.m. on a cold Thursday night. My cousin, David, was pushing one of his twin brothers in a stroller around the kitchen. David's mother was washing, and David and I decided to make hot cocoa. When the water was hot, we put our cups on the table and poured the water. David began to push the stroller again, but when he turned around, he hit the table. My cup of burning-hot cocoa fell on his arm and scalded him. He was curled on the floor and yelling. The house was in a panic. Finally, the ambulance arrived. David's arm had a burn at least 3 inches long and 1 $^1/_2$ inches wide.

David is better now, but still has a scar on his arm for life. Ever since that accident, I have always been careful with hot drinks. I learned from this accident that you should never put hot things on a table with loose legs and should never put hot drinks near children. A small child could get very badly hurt or even killed. Please ask an adult to supervise children when they are around hot drinks.

Averill Kelley, 12
Stamford

Dr. Baker's Comment:

Many children are burned each year by hot liquids. Most of these accidents can be avoided. Averill's advice is good advice: Always be careful around hot liquids.

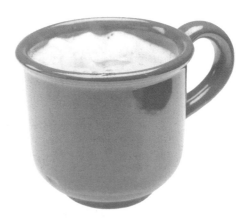

Chicken Turnover

One night, my sister Laura was baby-sitting for me and my other sister, Jocelyn. Laura was making chicken for dinner. When the chicken was done, Laura tried to take it out of the oven with one hand, but the pan flipped over. The grease and chicken fell all over Laura's right arm.

Dr. Baker's Comment:
Grease burns are common, painful, and dangerous. Take extra care in the kitchen. It is better to avoid burns than to have to treat them.

Laura was very badly burned. Her arm was red, and there were bubbles from her elbow to her wrist. We put cold water on her arm to wash off the grease and stop the swelling. Then, we put ice all over it to keep the swelling down and cool the burning. The next day, we had to take Laura to the doctor's. The doctor said she had a really bad third-degree burn. He gave her a special kind of ointment that she had to rub on her arm every couple of hours every day so that the burn would not get infected or scarred or hurt so much.

When you take hot food out of the oven, use two hands so you won't get burned like my sister did. Please take this seriously, because one day it might happen to you. If you do get burned, tell your parents and get medical attention right away.

Thomas Laudisi, 13
Bridgeport

Hot Stuff

When I was five years old, I was in my car with my brothers, my sister, and my father. I was in the front seat, and my brothers and sister were in the back. We were parked in a parking lot.

My father turned around to talk to my sister and brothers, not realizing I was fooling around with the cigarette lighter. I pulled out the lighter and touched it with my finger. It was burning hot, and soon I was screaming.

My father sped me to the emergency room. He later told me he went through three red lights. I yelled all the way there. At the hospital, a kind doctor soaked my finger in a liquid solution for about half an hour and then put medicine and bandages on it. For the next two weeks, my mother had to treat my wound twice a day.

Children should be taught that lighters are extremely dangerous and should never be touched. Better yet, adults with children shouldn't have lighters.

Cigarettes are bad for your health, anyway, so parents would be better off without them.

Shmully Levitin, 9
New Haven

Dr. Baker's Comment:

Shmully is right. Everything connected with cigarettes is harmful. Also, remember that it is always dangerous to touch any controls in a car or other vehicle. Large machines are meant to be operated by adults, not children.

Cars

A Miracle

I played in a football jamboree in Bristol. When it was time to go home, Andrew, one of the other players, stopped to talk to a friend, and his parents went ahead to their car. His parents were in a hurry and motioned for Andrew to follow them across the street. Thinking the coast was clear, Andrew proceeded to cross the street. Boom!

The driver put on the brakes, but the car still hit Andrew. Everyone could hear the tires screech and the force of the hit. Andrew was thrown several feet into the air and came down, head first, on the windshield.

He was lying in the road, and everyone rushed to him. He was bleeding from his ears, his head, and other parts of his body. Someone wrapped him with bandages and wet cloths. Others ran to nearby houses, banging on doors, asking for someone to call 911. A doctor who had been watching the game performed CPR on Andrew. [CPR stands for Cardiopulmonary Resuscitation. It is an emergency first-aid procedure used to restore a person's breathing.]

Soon, paramedics arrived at the scene. The Life Star helicopter took Andrew to a nearby hospital. The driver of the car was arrested. Everyone was horrified by what had happened and prayed that Andrew would pull through. The X rays later revealed that he had only broken his ankle. It was a miracle!

My advice to other kids is to be very careful when crossing roads. Look both ways. When you get your driver's license, don't speed! If your carelessness were to

Dr. Baker's Comment:

Jeremy's story is a good example of how even parents can sometimes make mistakes.

Both Andrew and his parents were careless because they were in a hurry. If they had taken the time to be careful and watch for oncoming cars, Andrew would not have been injured. Now, they have all learned that it is worth the little bit of extra time and care that it takes to stay safe and healthy.

cause injury to someone, you would have to live with it
for the rest of your life.

Jeremy Godenzi, 13
Harwinton

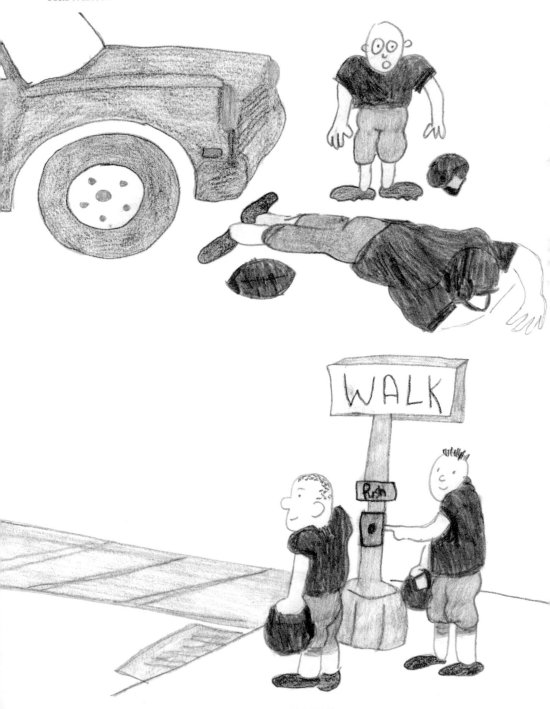

Runaway!

My mom, my four-year-old sister Erin, and I were going to the Verplank pool to swim. My mom was on the phone, and my sister got impatient to leave and got into the car. Somehow, Erin pushed a lever that made the car go down the driveway. My sister was scared, so she tried to stop the car by dragging her feet. It didn't work, and she was pulled out of the car. The car ran over her face.

My mom called 911 right away. The emergency team got to our house quickly, but they had to call the helicopter Life Star. They rushed Erin to the hospital, where she was in the intensive-care unit for one day and in the hospital for four more days. Erin fractured her skull and part of her shoulder. Lucky for her, she didn't have any lasting problems and got better soon.

Car doors should always be locked, and parents should not let little children near cars when they're not around to supervise.

Katie Mack, 11
Manchester

Dr. Baker's Comment:

Erin was fortunate to recover from her serious injuries. You are quite right, Katie. Parked automobiles should be locked, and children should not get into them unless they are told to by an adult. Most important, children should never try to operate the controls in an automobile or any other vehicle.

Buckle Up

Two years ago, one day before Thanksgiving, my mom was going to drive me and my brother, William, to school. It was very cold, and I couldn't open the car door because it was frozen shut. My brother got into the car and helped push it open from the inside. When Mom started to back the car out, she felt cold air. She turned around and saw that William's door was open. He hadn't slammed his door completely shut when he got in to help me, and when the car started to move, he fell out. William's hand got stuck under the tire. He was bleeding and all scraped up. We wrapped his hand in a towel with an ice pack and took him to the hospital. The staff there cleaned William's hand with soap and water and took X rays.

Andrew was lucky that his injury wasn't worse. If he had fallen a few inches closer to the tire, he could have injured his head instead of just his hand. We all learned a very good lesson. Always buckle up, no matter how short the ride. Check the doors and lock them—before the car starts to move—and never unbuckle your seat belt or open the doors until the car has stopped and is turned off. Okay?

Dr. Baker's Comment:

If Timothy or William had asked their mother to help with the frozen car door, they could have prevented William's injury. It is always better to ask for help from an adult when something does not work properly, rather than trying to fix it yourself.

Timothy Stobierski, 9
Ansonia

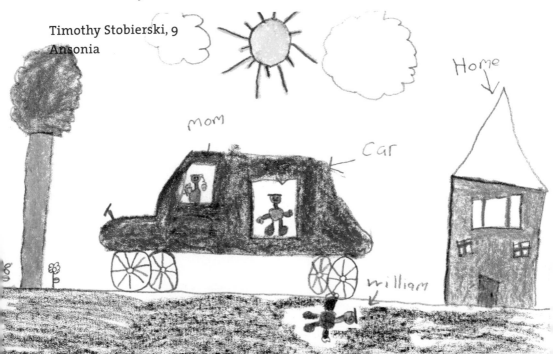

The Worst Kind of Driving Lesson

When I was five years old, my mother and I were at my friend's house. While my mother was chatting with my friend's mother, I took the keys for the van from my mom. She figured I was just going to play with them—but she figured wrong.

Dr. Baker's Comment:

Lauren was very fortunate. Many children are injured each year while trying to operate cars and other machines that only adults should operate.

Never turn on any machine unless you are asked to do so by an adult—and never try to drive a car or other vehicle unless you are trained and qualified to drive.

I got into the driver's seat and glanced over to find my sister in the passenger's seat. I jammed the key into the keyhole and turned the key, starting the engine. All of a sudden, I felt the car start to roll down the hill. I pushed on the gas pedal, and then pushed the brake pedal so suddenly that the sliding door went flying off the van. Suddenly, my mom was by the side of the van. As I pushed the brake pedal, my mom said, "Lauren, push that pedal again, and hold it!" As I did that, my mom said, "Turn the key to the left!" The engine stopped, and my mom gave a sigh of relief. If my mom didn't give me those instructions, I would have gone rolling into the trees. I put my sister's life in danger, along with my own. Now I know better. I will never drive a car again, until I'm old enough to learn how to do it the right way.

Lauren Wiley, 12
Bethany

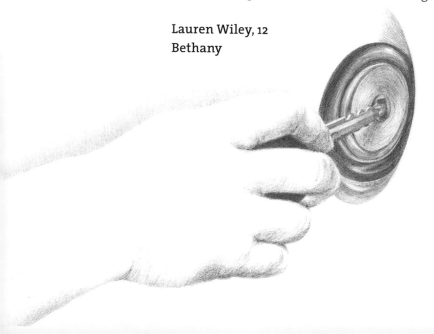

Chain Saws

Better Safe Than Sorry

My father wanted to cut down a tree in our backyard, so he got the chain saw from the basement. He stood on a ladder to cut the top of the tree while his friend held the ladder. Suddenly, the ladder shook, and my father lost control of the chain saw, which was still running. The saw cut into his forearm. My father jumped off the ladder, and his friend tightly wrapped a towel around my father's arm. He was taken to the hospital immediately. The next day, doctors performed surgery to connect severed nerves, arteries, veins, and tendons.

My father received physical therapy for several months. After the wound had healed a bit, he had to practice picking up small objects. He also had ultrasound treatment, which is the use of electron waves to stimulate nerve repair. He had daily hand- and finger-strengthening exercises to do at home.

If you work around the house, be very careful. If you need to stand on a ladder to reach high places, always make sure the bottom of the ladder is firmly planted on the ground. Also, always have someone nearby, both to support the ladder and in case of emergency. If no one had been there when my father was cut with the chain saw, he could have lost a critical amount of blood. So, be prepared, be alert, and most of all, be safe! Remember, better safe than sorry!

Celin Chacko, 15
Bridgeport

Dr. Smothers's Comment:

Celin, you're right. Better safe than sorry. Unfortunately, your father did not follow your advice. It's just not safe to operate dangerous tools like chain saws, hedge clippers, branch trimmers, or other sharp tools while standing on a ladder, on a roof, or in a tree. Anything can—and probably will—happen. Celin's father learned that the hard way.

Be smart. Always try to think of—and try to avoid—the worst thing that could happen.

Next time, I hope Celin's father will call a professional to cut down his trees.

Choking

Fear of Fireballs

I've been scared many times in my life, but never like this. I was in the fourth grade. Every day, while waiting for the bus, a few of my friends and I stayed after school to clean up my teacher's room.

She'd always give us candy. One day, after I cleaned the chalkboard, she gave me a fireball. I popped it into my mouth. Right after that, my bus came, and I ran outside. I sat in a seat next to Becky. I forgot that the fireball was in my mouth until Becky reminded me to throw it away. Just before the bus started moving, I stood up to ask the bus driver if I could throw the candy out. I lifted up my head, the fireball went back into my throat, and I began to choke.

The bus started moving slowly. I put my hands around my neck trying to breathe. Everyone was yelling, "She's choking!" and I heard Becky say "She's only faking!"

When the bus driver heard the yelling, she looked in her rearview mirror and saw that my face was bright red, almost blue. She slammed on the brake and ran to me. She pulled me into the aisle and started doing the Heimlich maneuver [a first-aid procedure used to remove an object from a choking person's windpipe]. Out popped the fireball. I felt so relieved to breathe air. I was so scared that I was going to die. All the kids were crying, especially my sister Ashley. The teacher who gave me the candy felt guilty, but I told her it wasn't her fault. She handed me a rose to help me feel better. I just wanted to go home and go to bed.

I had a sore throat for a few days. For about two or three months, I was afraid to eat anything because I thought that I was going to choke again. I wouldn't let my sisters or brother eat anything hard. I got so mad at them if they ate grapes, sucked on ice, or ate a fireball around me. Four years have passed, and I still have never forgotten this—and I have not touched one fireball since!

The bus driver, Lori Moir, was presented with a plaque for saving my life. I'm so thankful to her. If it wasn't for her, I probably wouldn't be here right now. She must have been so scared, probably even more than I was, but she was brave enough to help someone in danger.

DO NOT eat on the bus! Bus drivers don't say this to be mean. They say it for your own good.

**Amber Royce, 13
Portland**

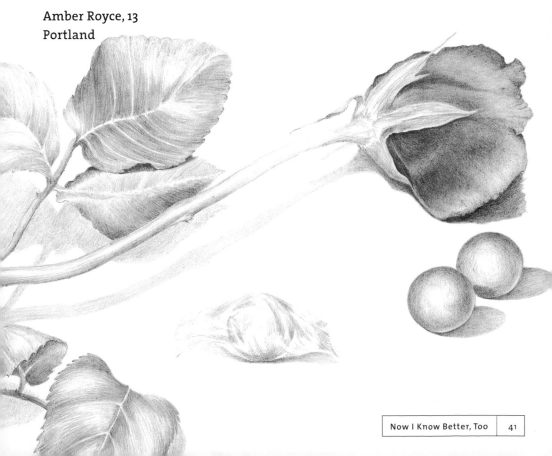

Not the Happiest Birthday

"Yahh, Mom, Dad! My throat!" I screamed, starting to cry. Those were the last words I thought I would ever utter.

Dr. Baker's Comment:

Justin, you were lucky to have someone nearby who knew how to get that ring out of your throat! The lesson here is to put only food in your mouth, and to chew that food thoroughly. Toys are just not meant to be tasted.

It was my 11th birthday. Everyone had left the party except for my mom, dad, and brother. My parents were downstairs, and I was upstairs playing with a ring from my goody bag. I put the ring in my mouth and swished it around. All of a sudden, it went down my throat. It was stuck, and I started trying to burp. I tried screaming for help, but all that came out were muffled, gurgling noises. I couldn't get the ring out, and I couldn't breathe. My mother yelled, "What's the matter?" I kept trying to tell her, but she couldn't understand me. I ran downstairs, throwing up water. My father used the Heimlich maneuver. He placed his arms below my rib cage and pushed up firmly. The ring finally came out, covered in blood. I was okay, but my legs were shaking.

I couldn't believe that I almost died because of something so careless and stupid. No matter how old you are, never put anything but food in your mouth. I was lucky that my dad knew the Heimlich maneuver, because if he didn't, I probably wouldn't be alive today. So, kids, don't put any type of object in your mouth and, parents, please learn the Heimlich maneuver.

Justin Robert Wentworth, 11
North Haven

Cuts

The Toy That Ate My Brother's Finger

During the third inning of one of my baseball games, my brother, David, came running across the field staring at his index finger. It was cut off to the first knuckle. He and his friend had been playing in the playground with a back-hoe toy. David had put his finger in the moving parts of the back hoe while his friend was pulling the levers that controlled the shovel.

My mom took David to the hospital. The doctors examined his finger and decided that David needed a special surgery called recuperative surgery. This is a type of surgery often used to treat a person who is severely injured. The doctors removed skin from one finger and sewed it onto the cut finger.

Don't put anything into the moving parts of a toy. Body parts can be cut off by the mechanism. Objects can break and hurt someone. I suggest that you always keep an eye out for trouble.

Jason Cote, 13
Burlington

Dr. Baker's Comment:

Jason is correct. Toys can often cause cuts and bruises, as well as more serious injuries like David's. Always be careful when playing with toys that have moving parts.

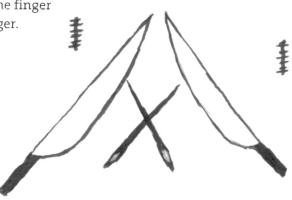

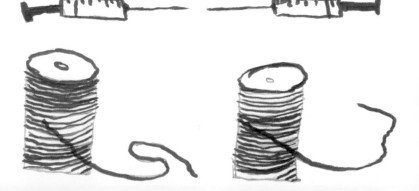

Not Kid's Stuff

I took my mom's scissors and was playing with them near my baby brother. He put his tiny finger in the way, and I cut his finger by accident. Blood went everywhere. He was screaming. My mom was very upset. It took a long time to stop the bleeding. My mom called the doctor, and he said if the bleeding did not stop to bring my brother in. But the bleeding finally did stop!

Don't ever put scissors near a baby.

Taylor Diane Hyde, 8
East Hartford

Dr. Kennedy's Comment:
Scissors are great tools, but there is a lot to learn about using them: how to hold them, how to carry them, how to cut with them, and, most important, how to keep the sharp edges away from our own or other people's fingers. Taylor's lesson is a good one to remember: Always keep scissors away from babies.

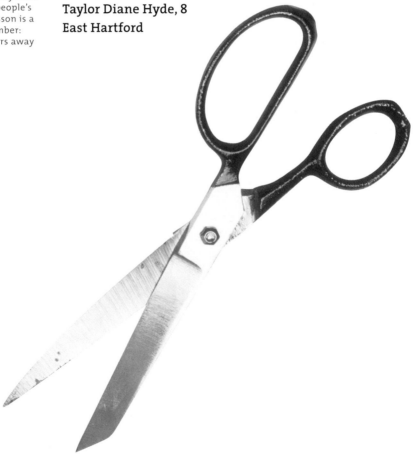

A Shattering Experience

My family and I were visiting my grandmother in Worcester, Massachusetts. I was five at the time, and my brother was two. My brother and grandmother were outside. From indoors, I saw my brother helping to water the garden. In a flash of jealousy (I liked watering), I ran out of the house. A full-length glass door led from the porch to the garden, and in my haste, my hand struck the door handle and my arm went straight through the glass.

The crash brought everyone running to find me hysterical and bleeding on the porch. My mother rushed me inside to wash my arm and wrap it in a towel. I remembering sobbing hysterically over and over, "Don't let me die!" As we drove to the hospital, my mother continued to assure me that I would not die. I was lucky, none of the glass was lodged in my arm. The doctors numbed my arm and stitched me up.

While I still bear the scars of the incident today, I was fortunate. Every year, millions of children in the United States sustain injuries that range from a minor abrasion to a trauma that results in death. The best advice I can offer to help prevent even one future tragedy is to use your head and take your time.

Greg Mulvey, 15
Guilford

Dr. Baker's Comment:
Rushing and carelessness often lead to injury. Greg learned that in a painful way. Hundreds of thousands of children are cut each year by glass or other objects. Take Greg's advice: Don't rush, take your time, and always think about what you are doing.

Don't Go There!

When I was two years old, I lost my left index finger. My mom and dad were in St. Thomas on a vacation, and they left my baby sister and me with a baby-sitter. I was playing outside near a running tractor that belonged to my baby-sitter's husband. He turned around to open the shed so he could put the tractor inside. I was curious about the spinning motor and decided to touch it. I stuck my finger into it and immediately began screaming. My finger had been cut off! Blood was everywhere! The baby-sitter rushed me and my finger to St. Mary's Hospital in Waterbury.

The hospital called my parents to tell them what happened. They were frantic. The doctors at the hospital didn't think they could reattach my finger. Doctors at Yale-New Haven Hospital said they could try, but I would be in surgery for about 20 hours and would need blood transfusions, and there was only a 10 percent chance that the surgery would work. My parents had to make a very tough decision not to have my finger reattached. They flew home on the next flight. I spent four days in the hospital.

Now I live with people always asking me, "What happened to your finger?" Every winter, when I wear gloves, people notice that I have a flimsy finger! The moral of this story is, never stick your fingers where they don't belong—especially in things that have motors!

Rachel Schiavone, 13
Old Saybrook

Dr. Smothers's Comment:

We hear stories like Rachel's far too often. Rachel shouldn't blame herself for her injury. Children are curious by nature. If adults—who know better—don't watch out for them, anything could happen.

Is your baby-sitter or relative watching you or your younger brothers and sisters as carefully as they should be? If you don't think so, tell your parents. You may help prevent some serious accidents.

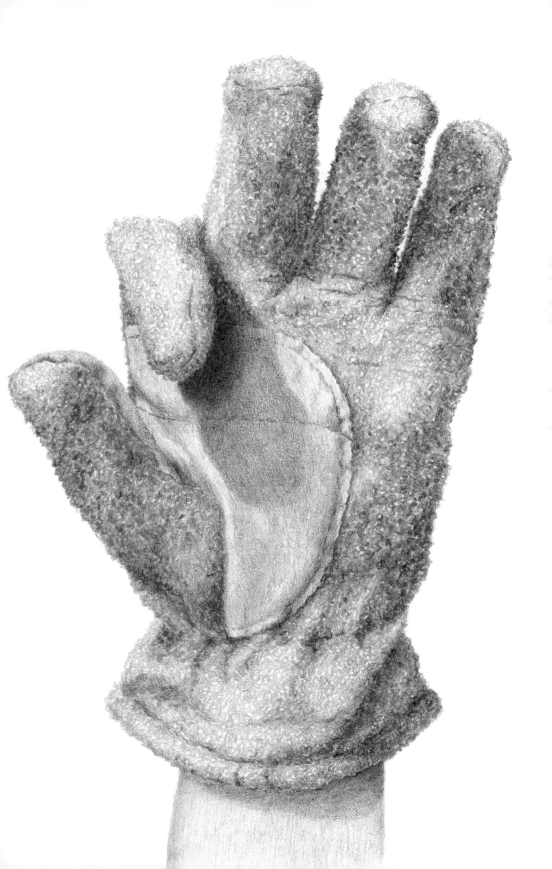

Ask for Help

One night, Mom and I were home alone. We decided to have dinner in the living room and watch the movie *The Jungle Book*. I wanted some chocolate milk so I went to the kitchen to get it. The container of chocolate milk was new and had a plastic seal on it. I couldn't open it, so I grabbed a knife and tried poking a hole in it. The knife slipped, and I sliced my thumb open.

Dr. Baker's Comment:
Daniel learned a valuable lesson. Knives are useful tools, but, like any other sharp instrument, they can also be dangerous. If Daniel had asked his mother for help, he could have avoided this injury. The next time you are having trouble with any task, ask an adult for help.

There was blood everywhere. I screamed for my mom, who came running. There was so much blood she couldn't even tell where I cut myself. She grabbed a towel and wrapped it around my hand. Then she got her keys and drove to Med-Now—very fast. When we got there, I was crying and freaking out. I was shaking so bad that they couldn't hold my hand still to look at it. I asked them to hurry up because all the blood that was coming out was scaring me. Finally, they cleaned the cut and stitched and bandaged my thumb.

To this day, I still have a scar to remind me of what happened. If only I had called my mom to open the container, this accident would have never happened. The lesson I learned was never use a knife to open anything. If you can't open it yourself, ask someone who can.

Daniel Alan Ritchie, 13
Stratford

Dogs

Keep Out!

When I was going into the kitchen one day, I noticed that my dog Hunter had taken something out of the garbage. I wasn't sure what it was, but I decided to try to take whatever it was out of his mouth. Then I saw that it was a huge chunk of roast beef. I didn't want him to choke on it, so I put my hand into his mouth. Then he bit me. But he didn't mean it. He was chewing and didn't know that my hand was in his mouth.

I screamed for my mom, and when she came in, she saw blood all over the place. My dog sniffed the blood and then went into his house. He knew he had done something bad. My mother and grandfather brought me to the emergency room at Bridgeport Hospital. My mother said I might have to get a tetanus shot [a shot to fight a type of infection known as tetanus], but because all my shots were up-to-date, I didn't need one. The puncture was deep enough to have 10 to 12 stitches, but the doctors said they don't stitch dog bites because they might seal in an infection.

It was hard to do many activities after that. Now, a couple of months later, I still am not able to feel my finger. I have to go to a specialist every once in a while.

My advice to you is, don't be dumb and try to take meat out of a dog's mouth when it is halfway down his throat. Call an adult to handle the situation. I am sure whoever it is will figure out something so that the dog doesn't choke.

Candice Loughman, 13
Trumbull

Drinking

Liza's Dreams

On August 29, 1997, my sister, Liza, was hit head-on by a drunk driver. The engine of her small car was practically sitting on her lap. The drunk driver tried to get Liza out of her car. The witnesses to the accident came over to her as soon as possible. The drunk driver told them that they were both fine and that they didn't need help.

Some of Liza's injuries were a broken hand, torn ligaments in her thumb and wrist, internal bruising, a broken rib, deep lacerations, dislocated knees, and post-traumatic stress. Liza was brought by the Life Star helicopter to the hospital where she stayed for 24 hours.

My sister almost died because of a drunk driver. How would you feel if you almost killed an innocent person because of a wrong decision you made? Your wrong decision would not only affect the victim but the victim's family and loved ones as well. I am telling you—as a kid and as someone who has experienced this—PLEASE don't drink. And when you get older, please don't drink and drive. Drunk driving can destroy dreams.

Hillary Ganoe, 13
Harwinton

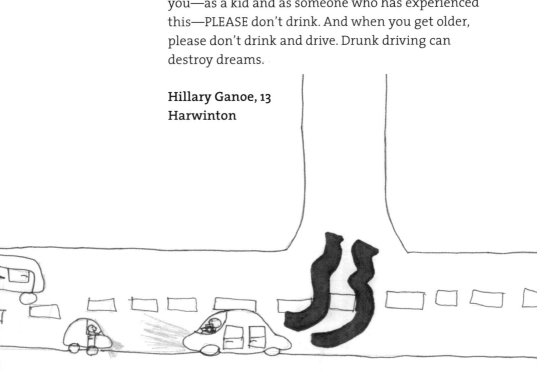

A Hard Lesson for Everyone

My twenty-two-year-old brother Eric was driving home late one night. He had been out partying and drinking. While he was driving down Route 30 he fell asleep at the wheel and crashed his car into a telephone pole. The Life Star helicopter soon arrived and brought him to Hartford Hospital. He had suffered a Traumatic Brain Injury (TBI) and, one month later, he was transferred to Gaylord Hospital (in Wallingford). Eric spent the next four years of his life in the hospital and had to learn how to do almost everything over again. Now, almost six years later, he still has trouble controlling his anger.

The point of this story is to tell you all how one careless mistake can change your whole life. Eric lost four years of his life. He is now living in an apartment in Meriden, working on holding down a job and getting his license back. His accident affected the rest of the family, too. There were costly hospital bills to pay. Visiting him so much, I literally spent almost half my life in a hospital.

Drinking and driving does affect you, and does affect others. Because of my brother's hard lesson, my whole family now knows better than to drink and drive.

Stacy Ridel, 13
Vernon

Dr. Kennedy's Comment:

Alcohol abuse is a tragedy—not only for the abusers themselves, but also for anyone who is unlucky enough to be involved in the accidents they cause. Children should make a firm commitment NOT to drink while they are under the legal age. Adults should make a firm commitment NOT to drink and drive—before they consume any alcohol at all. No one who drinks and drives thinks that he or she will be the one to cause an accident—but, sadly, experience shows that these people are often very wrong.

Drugs

You'll Never Miss It

We all make mistakes in our lives. Unfortunately, there is no way to go back and change the things that we've done, no matter how much we want to. I did one thing that I am particularly sorry for that will stick with me forever.

Dr. Kennedy's Comment:
More than 10 years ago, First Lady Nancy Reagan promoted the slogan, "Just Say No!" This advice is so easy and clear, but for so many, it is very difficult to follow. Please listen to Josh's message. You won't regret it.

I had started smoking marijuana as a pastime, and one morning, I passed out in my math class and ended up in the hospital. Later on, I found out that I came closer to dying than I ever wanted to at my age. I had never felt so ashamed and sorry in my life. I was not only sorry for me, but for my parents who I had let down even though they tried so hard to keep me away from drugs.

Besides feeling bad overall about what I did, I had other consequences to face. Because I was intoxicated in school, I was suspended for two weeks, which had a terrible long-term effect on my grades. Everything that I hoped would be so perfect was all being slowly destroyed.

This didn't have to happen to me, and it doesn't have to happen to anyone else. All you have to do is stay away. Never even pick up a joint or any other form of any drug. Just don't ever touch it, and you will never miss it. I'm not a cop or a parent or another adult writing a boring speech. I am a kid. I am a sixteen-year-old kid here telling you that I know drugs don't work, from my own experience. They almost ruined my life, but now I know better. I hope you do, too.

Josh Cacopardo, 17
Guilford

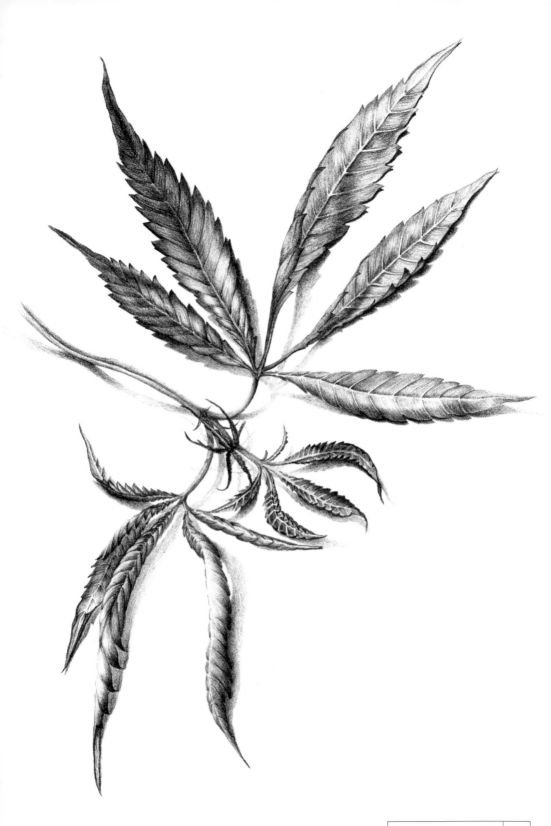

Eyes

Dr. Kennedy's Comment:

Our vision is a very precious thing. It lets us see smiles on the faces of the people we love and appreciate the beauty of nature. Injuries to our eyes can happen suddenly, while we are doing something that, under normal circumstances, we would not consider as being a threat to our eyesight—for example, hitting a golf ball in an open area.

In any activity, if there is any chance of a small object hitting our eyes, we should wear goggles or another type of eye protection.

Be Prepared!

I was about two years old, and my mother was folding freshly washed clothes. I was playing with different things, including a wire hanger. My mom turned her back for just a minute to get another article of clothing. Suddenly, I started to cry. Mom turned around to find me trying to pull the hanger out from under my eyelid. I still remember the lights and sirens as we pulled into the entrance of Bridgeport Hospital. The doctors and nurses removed the hanger from under my eyelid and gave me medication to stop the pain.

After this accident, I learned not to play with hangers or other dangerous objects that could hurt other people or myself and learned not to put things in or near my eyes. I also learned to watch young children closely because they get into the silliest accidents—and some of them can cause serious injuries or even be fatal.

I am grateful to my mom who knew how to react to the situation by calling 911. All baby-sitters and parents should know emergency safety procedures, such as CPR [Cardiopulmonary Resuscitation] and the Heimlich maneuver. Be prepared! That is what I learned from my experience and is the advice I would give to others.

Marcie Foulke, 12
Stratford

Ricochet!

One of the most serious accidents I've ever heard about was when a high school senior named Jamie got into trouble with a golf ball. Jamie was practicing his golf swing around his house and he hit the ball very hard. It ricocheted off the edge of his pool and hit him in the left eye. He had to be rushed to the hospital.

Jamie was in a lot of pain, but when he found out that the doctor had to remove his eye completely he was even more upset. If the doctor had left the damaged eye in, it would have affected the vision in Jamie's other eye. For weeks, Jamie had to wear a cloth pad over his eye to protect it. Then, he had to wear special glasses. The glass over his damaged eye was shaded to protect that eye from light. Although his artificial eye looked and felt the same, Jamie would only be able to see out of his right eye for the rest of his life.

The advice that I would give is that you shouldn't play with anything carelessly. Practice your golf swing in a place where there aren't any walls or sharp edges that the ball could hit and come back at you. If you are hitting a ball around your house, it would be safer to use a whiffle ball.

Jenna Petrucelli, 13
Shelton

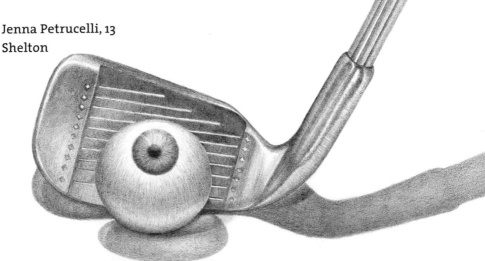

Age Doesn't Matter

My situation was rather silly. You would think I would know better.

One day, I was trying to unclog a container of a strong superglue. Suddenly, it squirted right in my eye! I screamed in great pain. It was burning my eye! My vision started to blur. I didn't know what to do. I was so scared. I thought I would be blind forever. That could prevent me from doing many things, even sports! I couldn't live without sports!

Quickly, I called my mom. She told me to wash out my eye. So, I stuck my eye under the faucet and let the cold water run on it. It just wouldn't wash out. My vision was still blurred! I waited to see if it would get better. It didn't, so my dad took me to the emergency room. There, they took a weird rinsing contact that was connected to a long tube and put it in my eye. The tube was connected to a big plastic bag that was filled with a cleaner liquid. I had to sit in pain for 45 minutes while the fluid cleaned my eye. For a week and a half, my eye was half closed because it was so irritated. My doctor said I could have gone blind if I waited any longer.

I was eleven years old then, but it just goes to prove that we need to be more careful about what we do at all ages. Age doesn't matter. Please be careful.

Marlene Rispoli, 14
Vernon

Falls

Maybe They Do Know Better

We used to live next to the woods, and my brother and I always used to go exploring. One time, we found two trees leaning on each other—one vertical and one horizontal. The vertical tree had little sticks coming out of it, like a ladder. My brother showed me how to climb it, with some help. I thought it was really cool.

The second time we went there, it had just rained. My father warned us not to climb the tree because it might be slippery. But totally ignoring my dad's words of caution, my brother and I headed toward the tree. When we got there, I saw that the tree was indeed wet and slippery. As I climbed, I realized I had nowhere to put my foot. I slipped, and a stick pulled up my shirt. I fell down almost the whole tree, sticks scraping my bare stomach the whole way. I started screaming. I had a huge cut across my stomach, and my white turtleneck was soaked with blood.

My brother let me ride home on his back. Thinking this was cute, my parents recorded us on the video camera. But when I climbed down, they saw my shirt. I had to take a bath and put soap all over my cut. It hurt! We put an antibacterial ointment on it, too. It took a long time for the cut to heal, and I still have a scar today, about five years later.

My advice to anyone is, listen to your parents. Maybe they've been through the same thing.

Danielle Amenta, 13
Portland

Dr. Kennedy's Comment:
It is not very surprising that Danielle slipped and fell while climbing that wet and slippery tree. It is also not very surprising that her advice to you is to listen to your parents. She would have been much better off if she had done that in the first place.

Copy Cats

Last summer, my brother and I learned a lesson about bad decisions. We were playing outside, climbing with bungee cords. A kid in the neighborhood had given us the idea. We were using the kind of bungee cords that you use to hold stuff on your bike. They had two metal hooks on them. My brother hooked the cord onto a piece of playground equipment. When he jumped, the hook snapped because it couldn't hold his weight. The cord smashed my fingers real hard and ripped the skin open on his chest. We were really scared. He had to go to a plastic surgeon and get 12 stitches. I thought my fingers were broken, but the X rays showed that they were just badly injured. We were really lucky that the hook didn't hurt our eyes or scar our faces.

We learned that to climb with bungee cords, you need professional equipment and adults who know what they are doing to help you. We also learned not to do things other kids tell you to do if you think it could be dangerous. Check it out with your parents before you do anything that could hurt you.

J.P. Culligan, 10,
and Danny Culligan, 8
Woodbridge

Dr. Kennedy's Comment:
Many people would question the wisdom of any type of bungee jumping or climbing, even by professionals with the proper equipment! J.P. and Danny know that they were very lucky. They also learned an important lesson: Don't copy what you see on television or feel pressured to do anything just because someone suggests that you do it, especially if it can be dangerous.

Neatness Counts

I have had more accidents than you could ever think of, but I'd say the scariest one was when I fell through a glass table. It was only a few feet to the floor but it felt like miles. After I fell, I noticed that I had tripped over my brother's train set. I had just enough strength to climb upstairs, tell my mom what happened, and get in the car. I went to the hospital. I had nine stitches. Eight were on top, and one was underneath my skin.

To this very day, the one underneath the skin is still there. I also had an X ray to find glass pieces. Then, the doctor gave me novocaine to numb the pain and checked my gash for glass. It all took three hours.

Having my mom next to me, I felt on top of the world. I didn't feel a thing. Later, I had to wear a splint that looked like a cast to keep my wrist from bending and opening the wound.

The lesson I learned is, always listen to your parents and do what they tell you. Now you know why they tell you to clean your room. Never leave your toys lying around. And while you're at it, make sure you brother and sister don't either.

Dave Kramer, 13
Burlington

Dr. Kennedy's Comment:

Even though Dave cut himself badly enough to need stitches, everything turned out okay. His mother and the doctor who treated him knew just what to do to make him feel better.

Knowing that we are well cared for can make all of us feel better—even if we have to make a trip to the hospital.

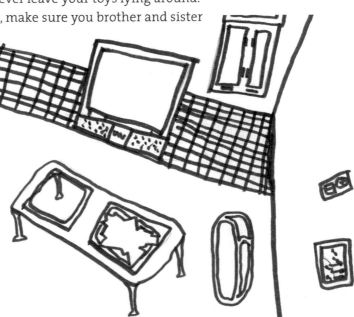

My Brother, Superman

When my brother Jeremy was five years old, he was obsessed with Superman. One afternoon, my mom was at work, my dad was working at home, and the baby-sitter was watching Jeremy for a while. Jeremy was wearing his Superman outfit of red tights, a Superman shirt, a cape, and Superman underwear. He was jumping on the bed, pretending to fly, and got too close to the edge of the bed. I bet you can guess what happened next. CRASH! Jeremy's little head was no longer bobbing up and down in the air. It was on the floor and bleeding. He had hit his head on the radiator.

Dr. Kennedy's Comment:
Bouncing up and down, whether on a bed or a trampoline, can be very dangerous because of just what happened to Jeremy—the jumper can jump right off the edge and hit someone or something. Beth's advice is as solid as a good mattress.

The baby-sitter ran to my father, who went crazy, which really scared Jeremy, who was already crying hysterically on the floor next to the sobbing baby-sitter. My dad immediately called my mom, who was calm and told Jeremy it was okay, but that he needed to go see a doctor. Jeremy calmed right down once he saw that my mother wasn't running around the house screaming and pulling out her hair (my dad wonders why he is going bald). My brother went to the hospital and got six stitches on his head. He also got my mother's lecture about how he is never to jump on beds again.

The advice I give is make sure your child knows that cartoons are cartoons and Superman can't really fly.

Beth Maco, 14
Stratford

Skating into a Boxing Ring

When I was four years old, my mom and I went grocery shopping. She had to use the restroom. I was bored while waiting for her. The floor was wet, and a paper hand towel was on the floor. I had a great idea! I would skate on the paper towel while I waited. Well, that didn't last long. I fell smack on my face and let out a scream that would wake up the dead. My mom rushed out of the stall. My nose was swelling, and blood was everywhere. We rushed out of the restroom. Guess who was also shopping? A paramedic on duty. He had his rescue truck outside. He radioed an ambulance to come and get me. The paramedic put an ice pack on my nose while we waited.

At the emergency room, they took X rays of my nose to see if it was broken. It wasn't, but I had two black eyes to go with my swollen nose. My advice to other kids is, do not play on wet floors—unless you want to look like you came out of a boxing ring with Mike Tyson.

Angie Mavrakis, 10
West Haven

Dr. Kennedy's Comment:
Not all falls and injuries occur while climbing. Angie's story reminds me of the advice of lifeguards at the pool in the summer: "Walk, don't run!" Wet surfaces are slippery, whether by the pool or in the supermarket. Even walking across them requires careful attention.

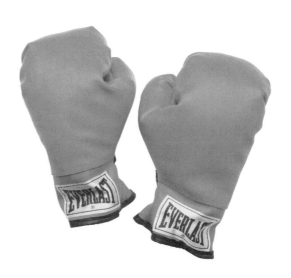

Upside Down and—Splat!

When you're a kid, you do some interesting things.
I thought, if I could do cartwheels on flat land, why
couldn't I do them on anything—or should I say
off anything.

In the front of my old house, there was a wall that was
about a foot above the ground. I thought it would be
really cool to do a cartwheel off it. The first time I tried
it, I was okay. I tried it again and still I didn't get hurt.
At this point, I thought I was a pro. My mom told me
to stop before I got hurt, but did I listen? No. I kept
cartwheeling off the wall. If you could do it once or
twice, then obviously you think you can do it again.
I tried my amazing stunt one more time, hit the stone
wall, and fell flat on my face. When I got up, my left

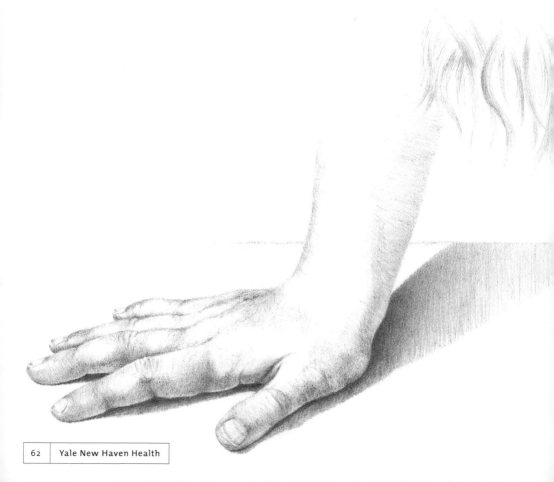

eye was scraped and bleeding. The entire left side of my face was skinned, and there were little pebbles embedded in my forehead. I was screaming and crying, and all I could hear was my mom saying, "Vicky, what did I tell you? I told you, you were going to get hurt, but did you listen? No!" My mom was hysterical, and she didn't know what to do.

The next day, I woke up and I looked at myself. It was terrible. My eye was swollen shut, and I had a bunch of scrapes on my face. I wish I had listened to my mom.

From that day on, I learned my lesson. I now understand my mom was only telling me to stop cartwheeling off the wall because she didn't want me to get hurt. If you're in the same situation, and feel you want to be defiant, stop and think, "Is it really worth getting hurt?"

Victoria Marrus, 14
Wallingford

Dr. Kennedy's Comment:

Victoria's advice is absolutely correct. Children often don't realize that their parents give instructions because they are trying to save them the tears and pain of an injury. Victoria's mother did not want to spoil her fun—she just wanted to prevent her from getting hurt while doing something dangerous, like cartwheeling off a wall.

Whenever you decide to try something that seems like fun, think about the risks of getting hurt—and make the wisest choice.

The First Time

My name is Kayla, and I'm sorry about what I did.

Five years ago, my brother Jordan, our friend Eric, and I were playing. We were climbing a ladder to the second floor of Eric's house. Eric's parents told us many times not to climb the ladder, but we didn't listen—and yes! someone finally got hurt. My brother was more than halfway up the ladder when he slipped and fell. We heard a small scream, then a BANG! on the pavement. I looked down and screamed. Jordan was on his back. He was not moving. Eric and I picked him up and put him in our toy jeep and drove him through the woods back to our house. I was yelling and trying to tell Dad the story, but it took him a couple of minutes to understand me. Then, he saw Eric and the jeep coming.

Dr. Kennedy's Comment:

It's fun to climb up high and look down. The problem is that sometimes the fun of looking down is spoiled by falling down.

Before you head up a ladder, have an adult stand at the bottom to hold and steady the ladder. Then, if you slip and fall, the adult can catch you—and you'll avoid an injury like the one Jordan suffered.

Jordan was rushed to the emergency room for X rays. There was a crack in his skull. They had to keep him awake all night long, because that is how they treat a concussion [an injury to the brain].

Jordan was badly hurt and stayed in the hospital two days. When he left, he was okay. It could have been much worse. I felt terrible, like it was all my fault. Jordan was very lucky, but not all kids are as lucky as he was.

Kids, listen. Someone might get hurt, maybe not the first time, but eventually, like my brother did. Please listen to adults—the first time.

Kayla Perruccio, 12
Portland

Firecrackers

PHSSSSSS....

One sunny morning, my three friends and I stopped at the gas station and bought firecrackers. We bought smoke bombs and poppers. I don't know why I bought them—for the sound, the noise, or the colors—but I do know that what happened that day was a surprise.

My friends and I went the small lake next to my house. We lit the first firecracker, and it made a sound that went PHSSSSSS. The sound and colors it made were cool. We lit all of the firecrackers, but there was one special one left. It was in a shape of a tree, and I wanted to light it so badly. I turned the lighter on, but then I saw my mom's car. I quickly put the firecracker in my pocket without thinking. Then I heard a noise in my pocket. All of a sudden, my pants started burning. I grabbed the firecracker and threw it away, but it was still going. I still remember that. It hurt so badly. My skin was burning and bleeding. Mom ran, saw that I was hurt, and quickly took me home and gave me medication to ease the pain. I felt horrible. Two hours later, I was lying in my bed thinking. I couldn't move my leg. I thought about how stupid I was to put that firecracker in my pocket. Now I'm 13, and I have learned to be cool about fire and to light fire only with adults around—or wait until I'm 18.

Paul Boho, 13
Stamford

Dr. Kennedy's Comment:
Paul is right. Fireworks are cool. They're fun to watch, and it's great to listen to their big booms—but they are also very dangerous. They can cause serious burns, damage our sight or hearing, or cause terrible injuries to hands and limbs. That is why most firecrackers are illegal to buy and use in many states—and that is why on special occasions, like the Fourth of July, town officials hire professionals to set off the firework displays for all to see and enjoy safely.

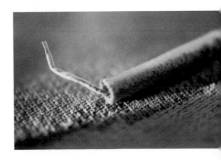

Goofing Around

Splish, Splash, Crash

There was a beautiful full moon that night. I was four years old and taking a bath with the help of my mother. When she was done, she told me to stay still in the tub until she came back with a towel. When she left, I decided to disobey her. I started to splash a little in the water. Splash, splash, splash. You could hear the waves of the splashing water. Circling around in the water, I got dizzy. Still dizzy, I tried to get up and slipped. Bang! I hit my right eyebrow on the rim of the bar on the shower door and the bathtub. My mother came back with the towel and screamed. Blood was all over me, in the water, and on the bathtub.

My mother rinsed all of the blood off me, then she put on my pajamas and gave me a rag to put on my cut to keep me from bleeding a lot. We got into the car and headed straight to the hospital. The doctor put me to sleep and gave me stitches. I didn't feel a thing. When the doctor was done, we went home, and I went to bed.

Ever since then, I have never played in the bathtub again, especially because the stitches left a permanent scar. Serious things can happen if you play in the bathtub—accidents like the one that happened to me, or even worse.

Danita Askew, 13
Stratford

Dr. Kennedy's Comment:

Bathtub safety is very important: checking the water temperature before getting in, moving about slowly so that you don't slip, and having an adult close by when small children are bathing. Nonslip skids should be glued to the bottom of tubs or to rubber bath mats to keep people from accidentally slipping.

Splashing in the bathtub can be fun—but twirling around in circles should only be done in a big, open patch of grass, where there's nothing you can bump into or slip on.

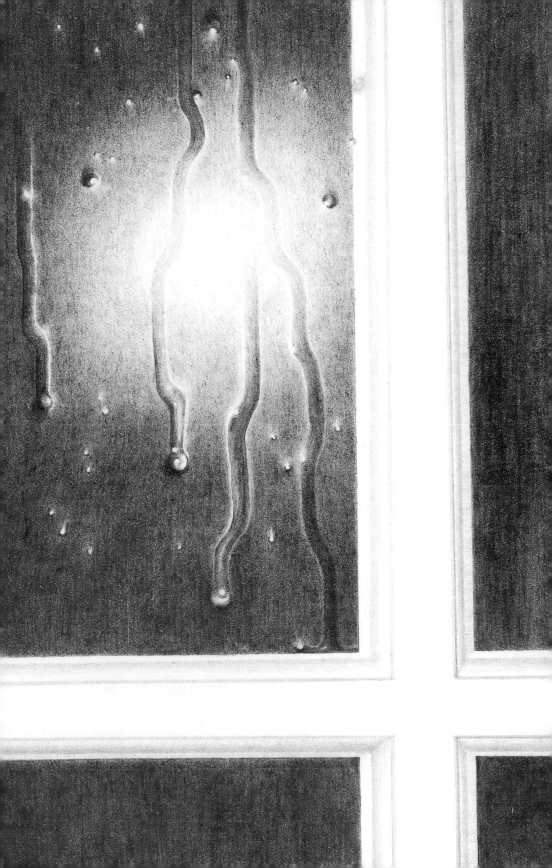

Running Blind

When I was eight years old, I was going home from my neighbor's house, and my six-year-old cousin, Caitlin, wanted to come, too. I told her that I would only let her come if she raced me. Of course, I knew I would win and then I could laugh in her face and rub it in. That was a typical eight-year-old thing to do. When I said "Go," I raced off.

My dad is a carpenter and always brings home junk from work. That night, he had brought home a metal rectangular stick with pointed edges. It was about 8 p.m. and dark. When I got close to my house, I ran faster and—BAM! I hit the metal stick. For the first couple of seconds, when I saw the blood, I was so shocked that I didn't feel anything. Then, the pain hit like a bullet. It felt like a saw had cut through my head. There was blood trickling down my face. By then, I was screaming bloody murder. My cousin was standing in front of me in shock. She had no clue what to do. I cried so hard I couldn't see. About two minutes later, my mom and our neighbor came running over to help me. The cut was from the corner of my eye to the middle of my neck. They said I was lucky, because if the cut had been any closer to my eye, I would have needed to have my eye removed! I had to wear a patch over my eye for a week until it healed. I still have the scar to this very day.

I advise that you always watch where you're going— and never run in the dark. You never know what lies ahead of you. The world is full of surprises.

Samantha Matson, 13
Vernon

Dr. Kennedy's Comment:

Samantha is giving us good advice. We should always watch where we're going, and when that is difficult to do—for example, at night when it is dark—we should go especially slowly and carefully. She is right when she warns us that "the world is full of surprises."

Toothless

When I was six or seven years old, I was running around in my grandma's kitchen. She told me to stop, but I didn't listen. I started to run faster and faster. Suddenly, I slipped, banged into the counter, and hit my teeth. After a few days, my tooth started to turn gray! My parents decided to take me to the dentist. When the dentist checked my tooth, he said I would have to get my tooth pulled out. So, a few weeks later, I went back to the dentist, and he pulled out my tooth. After that, I never ran around the house again. I also learned to listen to what my parents—and grandma—tell me.

Heather Lucas, 11
Ansonia

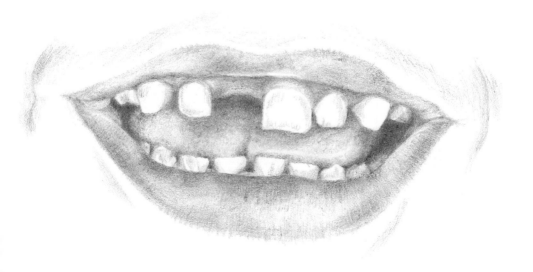

Quite a Mouthful

It was a typical Saturday morning, and everybody was busy getting ready for the day. My dad was in the kitchen cooking breakfast. Mom was in the shower, and my sister and I were chasing each other around the house. My mom could hear us running and yelled out "Stop running before somebody gets hurt!"

Dr. Kennedy's Comment:

Stairs are something we climb up and down all the time, and we don't give much thought to how dangerous they can be. Because we take climbing stairs for granted, we sometimes do careless things like run or try to carry too much up the stairs or trip on objects we've left there. Thanks for reminding us to slow down, Josh!

Too late. My sister fell while running up the stairs. She bit down so hard on her tongue when she fell that she cut it wide open. If she had bit any harder, she would have bitten half of her tongue right off. She started to scream, and blood was everywhere. My dad was upset and scared. He grabbed a roll of paper towels to sop up the blood and to slow down the bleeding as he and my sister ran out the door. My dad told my mom that he was taking my sister to the emergency room and to meet them there. My mom threw on her clothes and raced to the hospital. I stayed home, still dazed.

At the hospital, the doctor gave my sister some gauze and had her put pressure on the cut to stop the bleeding. After the bleeding slowed down, the doctor swabbed her mouth out to kill any germs. They called in a surgeon to look at her tongue to see if stitches would be necessary. Luckily, they were not. My sister had to eat soft foods, such as Jell-O and ice cream. By the next day, the hole had closed up almost completely.

My advice to you is not to run in the house, especially on the stairs. Don't stick out your tongue, either. It's disrespectful and can be dangerous. Boy, have I said a mouthful!

Josh Sinclair, 13
West Hartford

Guns

Jon's Terrible Mistake

"Bye, Jon! We'll be home later," said Jon's mom and dad. Jon, a thirteen-year-old boy who was my friend, went inside his house and heard on the radio that a famous musician committed suicide. Jon wanted to know who the musician was. He listened more and heard that it was a musician that he loved and idolized. Jon was so sad that he ran through his house, into one room and then into another, looking for something. He soon came out of one room with a loaded shotgun in his hands. Jon went onto the porch of his house and shot himself in the head. He committed suicide, just like the musician he loved had done. When his parents got home, they found him lying on the porch. He had a small funeral that my mom attended.

Dr. Kennedy's Comment:
Guns can kill. If there are guns in your home, they should be locked away. Each one should also have a trigger lock and should be stored unloaded. What happened to Jon was a terrible tragedy that could have been avoided.

Never play with guns and don't have guns in your house. Also, if you are upset about something in your life, you don't have to solve it by killing yourself. You can talk about what is bothering you with somebody and solve your problems in a different way. Finally, don't copy somebody else just because you like them.

Evan Kasowitz, 10
Orange

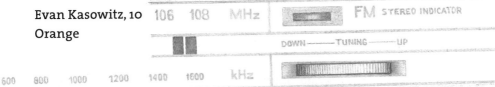

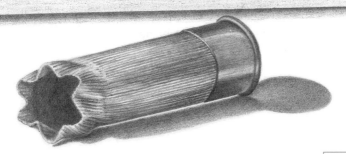

The 007 Wannabees

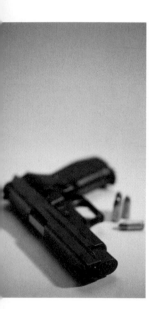

I'm a huge James Bond fan. I love fake cap guns and love to copy the stunts and spy moves I see in the movies. Last month, I was visiting my friend Spencer in New York. We had an hour before I had to catch the train home to Connecticut. Spencer said, "Let's go to a great store I know. We could get a fabulous cap gun there." He was right! The store was great—the cap-gun collection made my jaw drop. We each bought a gun, and when we got back to Spencer's apartment, we whipped out our guns to play spy. We didn't know a neighbor across the hall had seen us enter the apartment! I thought it would be cool to draw our guns on Spencer's dad as he came up the stairs to the apartment—but I figured someone might see us and get scared, so we didn't. That was the smartest decision I ever made.

Moments later, there was a knock on the door. We opened the door, but no one was there. Suddenly, three New York Police Department cops started screaming, "Come out with your hands up! Get up against the wall!" They all had their guns drawn. They screamed, "Where are the guns?" They frisked us roughly. I was scared! I could hear my heart pounding in my ears. Spencer kept saying, "They're fake, they're fake." After what seemed like an eternity, the officers checked out the toys and left saying, "I hope you learned a lesson."

Luckily, we learned the lesson before tragedy struck. The police can't take chances. Don't you take any chances either. Don't play with toys that look like real weapons. Because of a game, you could be shot—or even killed!

John Weselcouch, 13
Fairfield

Horses

Spooked!

My horse, Buddy, a black Tennessee Walker, quickly trotted down the stone path of Whitworth Farms to the outdoor ring. It was so warm, I could smell the sun-baked grass and see the heat shimmering from the ground. I loved riding, but this was nerve-racking. This was only my second time outdoors, and I was terribly nervous that I was going to make Buddy crazy, because horses scare easily.

My father was leading Buddy down a swerving stretch of road. My brother, Timmy, and my sister, Alia, were supposedly walking their horses a safe distance behind. We finally stepped onto the soft dirt of the ring. "Yeaahh!" Alia screamed loudly enough to wake the dead as her horse sprinted in front of Buddy. "Aaaahhh," I yelled at ear-splitting volume as Buddy reared. I grabbed at the reins, which I had not been holding. I could not get a grip on them, and they slipped out of my sweaty palms and fell away from me. I slid from the slick leather saddle to the ground. I hit the back of my head, which was not protected by a helmet, on a rock and had a long, bleeding cut. I had no permanent injuries, but my head hurt constantly, and I had to stay in bed awhile.

This incident taught me always to wear a horse helmet when riding. If a rider doesn't wear one, there could be horrendous results. A person can even die from head injuries.

Amber Black, 13
West Hartford

Dr. Baker's Comment:
Wearing a helmet while riding bicycles, horses, motorcycles, or anything else is good advice. The most frequent type of serious trauma in children is head injury. Regardless of whether you are sitting atop a bike or a pony, a helmet should be atop your head.

Nails

Stay Sharp!

I had just gotten all the wood for my tree fort and was ready to start working. I carefully climbed the tree and hammered in the supports. When the base was firm, I started laying out the floor, which takes a steady hand and careful planning. I had put in the first three floorboards when my friend Mike popped out from the bushes. He asked what I was doing and wanted to help. He climbed into the tree, and I handed him a hammer and went back to work.

We talked as we worked, and I wasn't paying much attention to anything when I suddenly put my hand down on a nail. The nail went straight through my hand between my little finger and my ring finger. I started screaming at the top of my lungs, and blood was everywhere. Mike ran inside and told my dad what had happened. They both rushed out to help me. My dad carried me inside and washed the wound out thoroughly and applied some medicine. Then he wrapped my hand in a bandage and propped it up on a pillow. I stayed inside the rest of the day and did not move my hand at all.

By the end of the week, I had a big scar on my hand and a lesson I would never forget. Now, whenever I build anything or handle sharp objects, I pay close attention to what I am doing. I also make sure I always have someone with me in case I get into trouble.

Michael Schroeder, 14
Fairfield

Noses

Diving for Pearls

When my sister was three years old, my family and I were going to go to the Greek Festival for the day. As we were riding along, my sister peeled off a pearl that was glued to her sneaker. Because she did not know better, she stuck it up her nose. She took another pearl off her sneaker and stuck that one up her nose, too. I noticed that she was doing this and told my parents.

We pulled over to the side of the road. My mom looked at my sister's sneaker and saw that there were pearls missing. Then, she looked up my sister's nose to confirm my observation. We drove to the doctor's office, and my sister was taken into urgent care. A specialist was called in for the job. He had to use special instruments to reach the pearls. Finally, they were removed successfully. We were very lucky.

Never stick anything up your nose. You may have trouble breathing and could even die. I hope that after reading this, you will never do this to yourself.

Andrew Valente, 13
East Haven

Dr. Kennedy's Comment:
There is an old saying that we shouldn't put anything smaller than an elbow into our ears. That is also good advice for noses. As Andrew's sister has learned, it can be very difficult for doctors to retrieve the beads and other small objects that children get stuck in their noses. Use your nose to smell the flowers—not as a storage cabinet!

Playgrounds

A Swinging Summer

I was six years old, and it was the middle of summer. I jumped around excitedly when Mom said we could invite Jen over. Jen was a new girl I had met who was visiting her grandma. Then I said, "Let's go play on my swings!" We raced to the swings, and I won. We started to play on the seesaw when Jen turned to the monkey bars and asked, "Can you do the monkey bars?" I didn't want to be embarrassed in front of my new friend, so I said, "Of course I can! Can you?" I lied badly. I could barely reach the monkey bars from the top step. Yet, I didn't want her to know I couldn't, so I started to climb to the top. When I got to the top, I stopped. "I don't want to do them right now!" I cried.

"Come on! I want to see you do it!" So I proudly but reluctantly grabbed hold of the first rung and swung myself off the step. I hung there for a while until Jen said, "Switch your hands! Like a monkey!" I took one hand off to switch to the second, but that was enough for me. I couldn't hold myself with one hand and came

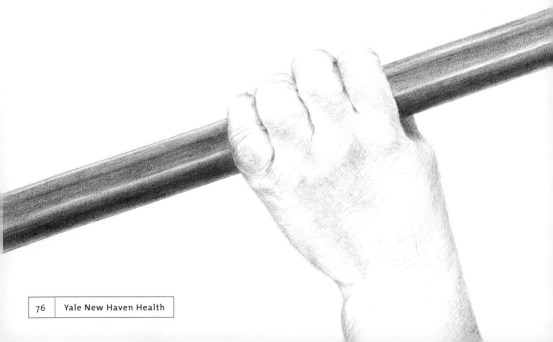

tumbling down. I landed on my left arm. I didn't move, but managed to say, "Get my mom!" Jen ran as fast as she could to my front door and knocked and knocked. When no one answered, she barged in, screaming,

"Help! I need help!" In the wink of an eye, my dad was standing in front of her. Before he asked who she was and why she was in our house, he said, "What's the matter?" Jen told him in two words, "Danielle's hurt." He ran outside and, after one look at me, he ran back in and told my mom to get ready to bring me to the hospital.

I was okay, if you don't count that itchy cast on my arm! But the next time, I won't show off for anyone if I know I can't do whatever it is they want me to try.

Danielle Albert, 13
Pawcatuck

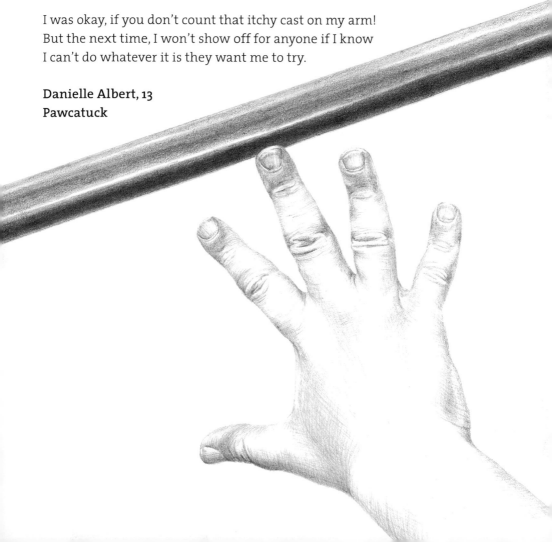

Slipping...

You know those metal swing sets, the ones with the swings and the slides? I used to have one, but my dad took it down. Why? Well, one summer, four years ago, my best friend, Amber, and I were playing on the swing set. My sister, Mackenzie, came outside. Mackenzie climbed the ladder to the top of the slide and began to run down. She slipped and grabbed at the bar on the top of the slide. What a big mistake! Her arm caught on a nail. Blood oozed out of the torn skin. I ran inside to get my father. He drove Mackenzie to the emergency room. She had to have seven stitches.

A few weeks later, my dad decided to take down the swing set. What happened to Mackenzie was an accident, but it could have been prevented if she hadn't been running down the slide.

If you run down slides, I hope that you'll stop.

Maureen Dunn, 11
Torrington

...and Sliding

"Never walk or run down the slide," my mother always told me—and she was right, as usual.

One night after dinner, when I was in second grade, I went down to the playground with my mom. I decided to show her that I could go down the slide running and standing up at the same time. Boy, that was a mistake! While I was going down, I slipped and fell on my bottom, but my left hand got caught between my body and the slide. I told everyone I was fine, but my wrist really hurt, so my mom took me back to our apartment and put a bag of ice on it. That made it feel a little better. I went to bed and said that my wrist was fine, which it wasn't—and I sure paid for that.

The next morning when I woke up, my wrist hurt a little bit. I went to school, and when my teacher looked at my wrist, it had swollen up more than it had been in the morning. My teacher took me to the nurse, who called my mom, and my mom picked me up from school and took me to the doctor. My doctor said that I had to get X rays. My wrist was sprained, and the doctor wrapped it.

After a few weeks, my wrist felt better. I learned two very important lessons within those weeks: Never go down a slide running or standing and try your best not to show off. Both of these lessons could keep you safe. I learned the hard way.

Danielle Palmer, 13
Stratford

Dr. Smothers's Comment:

You should always follow the basic rules of playground safety. Don't stand or run on slides, be sure there are adults nearby to supervise, avoid dangerous heights, and only play on safe equipment. Any sharp objects on playground equipment should be covered, and the ground should be cushioned with sand, wood chips, or rubber. Listen to Maureen's and Danielle's advice. Play it safe!

Big Mistake at Morley School

Dr. Kennedy's Comment:

This lesson regarding peer pressure is an important one, not only to help prevent accidental injuries like the one Kelly suffered, but also to avoid the bad decisions and mistakes that peer pressure can cause people of all ages. Knowing our own limits and abilities, knowing what we want to do, and knowing what is right should guide our decisions—not pressure from friends or others.

It was humongous. It gave splinters. It was...a playground? It was where everyone played at Morley School, but after my incident, I never trusted it. That day, my friends and I were showing off for each other. I decided to face my fears and perform the trick all my friends were trying and mastering. It sounds idiotic, but I was in the second grade, so I barely knew better. I hoisted myself onto the bar, straddled it, and started to ease over. All of a sudden, I sped up and zoomed around the metal bar. Somehow I had tilted myself, and my head was going to collide with the wooden pole supporting the bar! Students and teachers rushed to my side when I fell. They helped me up and brought me inside.

I almost fractured my cheekbone. Over the next four months, my left cheek turned the colors of the rainbow. My eye looked squashed, and the lumps on my face weren't too attractive.

All of this could have been avoided if I said to myself, "I don't think I am ready to do this yet." But I thought to be a grown-up meant taking chances. That was my biggest mistake. I caved into peer pressure and got hurt. My face has healed and so has my self-esteem. Now, if I feel pressured to do something, I can say no and feel good about myself.

The moral of the story is, if you feel pressured to perform an act that could hurt you and you don't want to do it, simply don't do it.

Kelly Curran, 13
West Hartford

Poison

Not Kid's Stuff

Four years ago, I was at my grandmother's house with my two brothers and two sisters. My brother Yaccov was two years old at the time. We were sitting around the table, and it was very quiet. My grandmother asked, "Where is Yaccov?" I said, "I don't know." We all became instantly worried about him because anywhere that Yaccov is, there is noise—but there was no noise. So I said, "I will go and look for him."

I went upstairs and checked all the rooms, and Yaccov was nowhere. Then I saw that my grandmother's door was open, so I decided to look in there, just in case he had ventured into her room. I saw Yaccov lying on the floor, and around him was a scattering of pills. I screamed, "Grandma, Yaccov is lying on the floor."

My grandmother ran up the stairs, and she realized right away that Yaccov had eaten my grandfather's pills. It was hard for my grandfather to open medicine bottles, so none of his medicine bottles were childproof. My brother had easily opened the bottle and had eaten the medicine. My grandmother's next-door neighbor rushed Yaccov to the hospital where the doctors pumped his stomach.

You should never eat medicine that is not yours, even if it tastes good and you think it won't hurt you. It will! One way that parents can prevent accidents is to have childproof caps on all medicine. Parents should explain to their children the dangers of taking other people's medicine. Also, medicine should not be left where it can easily be reached by children.

Chayala Avigdor, 13
New Haven

Dr. Smothers's Comment:

Chayala describes a very common and sometimes deadly accident. Many young children have serious accidents with their parents' or grandparents' medication. Chayala is right to remind parents that it is not always the child's fault. Parents should always keep their eye on children and keep dangerous objects out of any areas where children are likely to be.

Alarm in the Night

One night, as my family and I were sleeping, we were awakened by the sound of our carbon-monoxide detector. We called the fire department and were told to leave the house immediately. When the firefighters arrived, they opened all the windows and placed a large fan by the front door to let out the fumes. Then, they went around to each room checking the levels of carbon monoxide. They found that the fumes were coming from the furnace and advised us to call our heating company.

The serviceman arrived promptly because carbon monoxide is very dangerous. He found that one of the bolts that hold down the furnace cover was broken, which allowed the carbon monoxide to escape. He replaced that bolt and tightened the three other bolts. The firefighters checked the carbon-monoxide levels again, which were back to normal. We were then allowed to go back into our house.

If it had not been for our carbon-monoxide detector, my family and I would not have awakened the next morning. This is why you should have a carbon-monoxide detector in your home. Check it every month to be sure it is always working properly. Each spring and fall, when you change the time on the clocks, replace the batteries.

Meghan Borcino, 13
Naugatuck

Dr. Smothers's Comment:

Meghan, you are quite right. Carbon-monoxide detectors are very important. They are just as important as smoke detectors. For both of these devices, make sure you check the batteries or electrical connections on a regular basis. Perform frequent tests to make sure they are always working. Carbon monoxide is colorless and odorless, so you need the detector to determine its presence. By the time you feel sick, it may be too late.

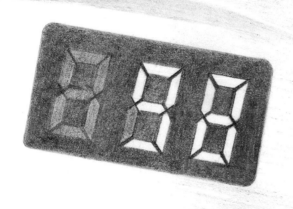

Carbon Monoxide DETECTOR

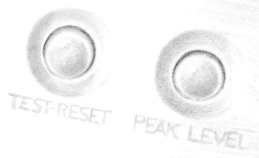

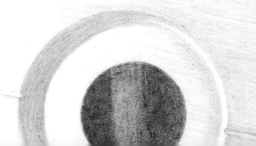

TEST-RESET   PEAK LEVEL

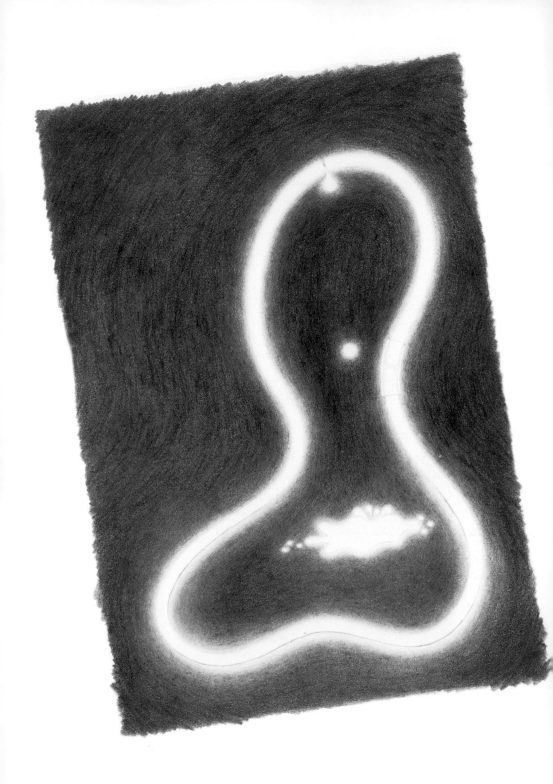

Squirt-in-the-Dark Necklace

Did you ever wonder what is inside a glow-in-the dark necklace? My best friend found out—the hard way.

I invited Colleen to a Bunnell Cavalcade. She agreed she would go and would sleep over my house that night. They were selling glow-in-the-dark necklaces there, and we both wanted one. One of the workers gave them to us for free! We were so happy.

Dr. Kennedy's Comment:

It's great to know how to help when accidents happen. Laura's advice to Colleen to rinse out her eye immediately was just right. Laura and her father made another wise decision when they called the Poison Control Center. I'm sure Colleen was very grateful for their help— and we thank them for their important advice for us.

That night, Colleen was lying down on the floor fiddling with the necklace. Suddenly, she started to panic, and I didn't know why until she stood up. The liquid from the necklace had gotten into her eye and leaked all over her. She started to cry. I quickly took action. I told her to go into the bathroom and rinse her eye with water, and went to find my father. I explained to him what had happened, and he called the Poison Control Center. The people there explained that Colleen had to rinse her eye for 15 minutes. If the burning didn't stop, we were to report back to them. Colleen was very tense wondering if she was going to go blind—but she didn't. Right now, she is fine, but we will always remember this accident.

The lesson to be learned is that even though something looks safe, it might not be. You think nothing could happen to you until it's too late. Just be aware at all times. Remember, if anything like this ever happens to you, a friend, or a family member, make sure that the person tells an adult what happened and calls the Poison Control Center.

Laura Sugrue, 13
Stratford

Running

Too Hot to Handle!

One hot summer day, my mom was running in the Torrington Blood Donors Road Race. After about 35 minutes, we saw her running down the hill to the finish line. My dad knew that there was something wrong. When she came through the finish line, her eyes were closed. She started to fall, and my dad caught her. He dragged her into a shady spot under a tree. Paramedics tried calling her name to see if she would answer. She just kept nodding every time they talked to her. They put her in an ambulance and went to the hospital.

The doctors put wet, cold washcloths all over her, but she was still unconscious. Her fever was 104 degrees. The doctor told my dad that when my mom woke up she would have something called "temporary amnesia and impending doom." She thought that she was going to die. My brother was scared because she kept screaming and thought that she had had a heart attack. The doctor gave her some fluids intravenously [through a vein] to calm her down and rehydrate [restore liquids to] her. After a while, she fell asleep.

The doctors at the hospital were upset because the road race had been held on such a hot day. It was 98 degrees that day, and the humidity was 100 percent. The advice I would give others is, don't run hard when it is really hot outside. When you're in a race, drink water at every stop where it is offered, and only run early in the morning or late in the afternoon, when it is cooler. Make sure somebody is always with you when you run.

Rebekah Prenoveau, 12
Harwinton

Dr. Smothers's Comment:
Rebekah accurately describes a very serious condition known as heat stroke. It can affect children just as easily as it did Rebekah's mother. All of her advice is right on the mark.

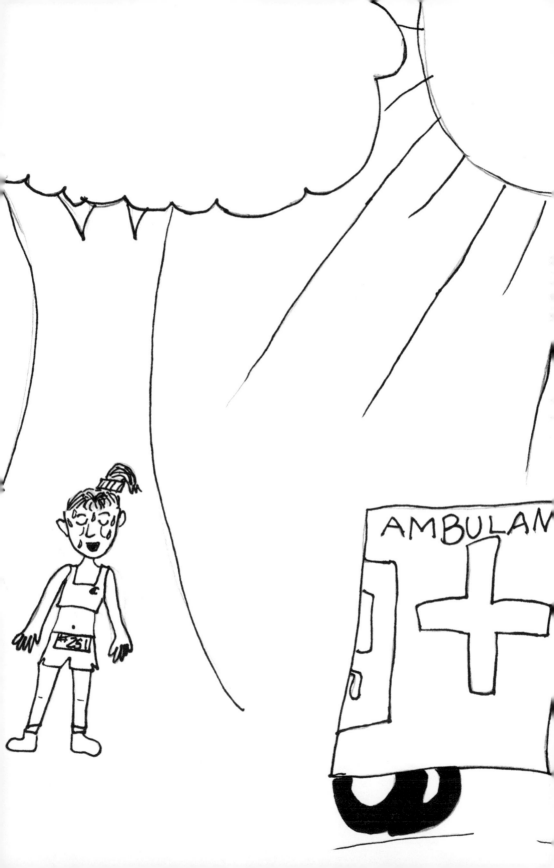

Skateboards

Flipped Out

Have you ever flipped off a skateboard? In September, I did. My friend was over, and we were taking turns on my skateboard. When it was my turn, I went down a big hill. I hit some gravel and sand, and my skateboard started to swivel back and forth. Eventually, I got thrown off. I landed head first on the tar, just missing somebody's mailbox.

I had cuts all over me—on my shoulder, wrist, both arms, both knees, and my foot. I could not move my arms or my shoulder without pain. Luckily, I did not have to go to the hospital. It took me two and a half weeks to recover, and I still have scars.

To avoid what happened to me, you should not go down a hill that is too steep. Do not ride a wobbly skateboard, especially on gravel and sand. Don't go too fast, or

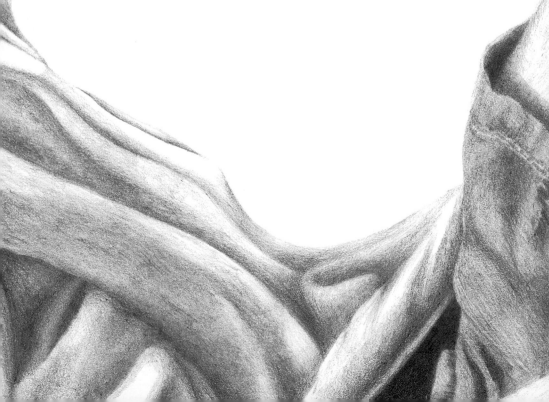

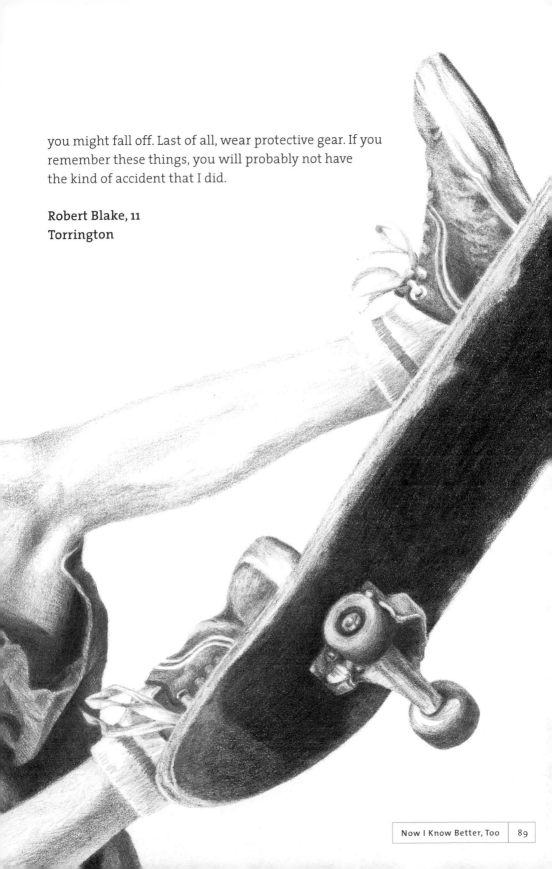

you might fall off. Last of all, wear protective gear. If you remember these things, you will probably not have the kind of accident that I did.

Robert Blake, 11
Torrington

Sleds

Out of Control

Your parents have probably screamed at you 100 times to wear a helmet, as well as not to fight on the stairs. Yes, all those things are important, but I have a new safety rule for you to consider. This rule deals with one thing that we all love to do in winter—sledding.

In March of 1993, my brother, Brendan, and I decided to go sledding. The snow had a thick, hard layer of ice over it, which made it very difficult to walk. We thought it was great because the sled could go much faster. The hill was extremely steep and ended at our house. Brendan hoisted himself up on the bright red, circular sled. It was brand-new, and he wanted to see how fast it went. He flew to the bottom. Then, something horrible and gruesome happened.

As Brendan got closer to the house, he started to scream, fearing for his life. When he opened his mouth, the solid ice acted as a knife and severed his tongue. It was literally hanging by a thread. That was not the worst of it. His bottom teeth ripped through his lower lip and left a jagged hole. Blood was everywhere. A surgeon had to stitch my brother's tongue back together. It took two hours, while I sat in the waiting room sweating bullets. Afterward, Brendan could barely talk, much less eat.

Please be more careful than we were. Make sure the path you choose for sledding does not lead to a house, wall, or street. If you find a good path, stamp it out with your feet or shovel so that you sled on snow, not ice. Always remember to use a sled that you can steer. Trash the circular sleds. You have no control over them even on powdery snow. Let my story be a lesson to you.

Eric DiPiazza, 14
Weston

Ice Isn't Always Nice

One very cold winter night, my mom, my brother, and I went sledding. We had so much fun! Someone had made a 5-foot-high jump out of snow. I decided to go down the jump. My mom told me it was not a good idea—but of course, I did not listen to her. I went down the hill and was moving faster than I wanted to. I hit a patch of ice and went flying off the jump. I flipped over and landed on my head. Then, the 20-pound sled landed on my freezing body.

My mom ran down the hill shouting. She took me straight to the emergency room. The doctor said that I needed an X ray. I heard my mom say that my stepmom and my dad were there, but I could not see anything. I had became unconscious. I soon regained my consciousness and told my parents that I loved them, just before I went to the X-ray room. When I came out, the doctor told my parents that I had a fractured neck bone plus two pulled muscles in my right arm. I needed to wear a sling and a neck brace. But I was okay!

There really is a lesson in all of this mess. The lesson is, listen to your parents. That may seem out of whack, but if I had listened to my mom, I would not have been in that situation. Please take what I say into consideration and listen to your elders. They really do know what's best for your safety!

Robert Warner, 12
Portland

Dr. Smothers's Comment:

Winter play is great fun, but as Eric and Robert now know, it can also be very dangerous. Almost all sporting accidents can be prevented. When riding a sled or snowmobile, always wear a helmet. Avoid steep hills unless there is a very long and safe flat area along them—and avoid going so fast that you lose control.

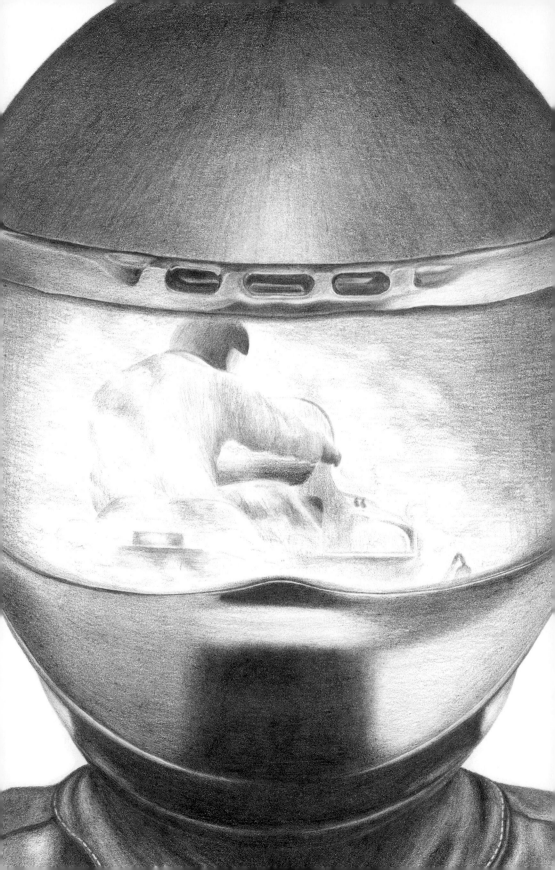

Snowmobiles

Wahoo!

"Wahoo!" I heard my buddy John say as we followed him. There were six of us: four family members and two friends. We all followed John because he had the fastest snowmobile. After we had lunch, there was a terrible windstorm, which blew snow all over. Even though we liked to ride, we waited awhile for it to settle—but it didn't, so we all headed home. I was on my new Jag Arctic Cat 650.

We went racing through the trails, skipping across ice, and winding around turns, when suddenly there was a blinding gust. If it wasn't for my helmet, I think the snow would have blinded me. We all stopped. We couldn't see the trail and didn't know what to do. John said, "This way," and took off, so we followed. As he sped up, we accelerated also, until suddenly we heard "AAAAH BAM." We all stopped. "Hey, where's John?" asked Joey.

John had gone off a cliff and into a pond, where we found him floating. We managed to get him out and found some help. John was rushed to the local hospital where he had surgery on his back. Today, he can't move his arms or his waist. He is still able to walk and talk, luckily. Doctors say he won't be able to move his arms for another six to eight years.

I still ride a snowmobile often, but I have a lot of advice to give. I would tell any rider to take precautions, ride only when it is safe, and always wear a helmet. Even though you are a good rider, accidents will happen.

Chris Cahill, 14
Bristol

Dr. Smothers's Comment:

John learned a hard lesson. Don't use snowmobiles where there are trees, fences, poles, big rocks, ponds, or lakes. When playing outside in the winter, you not only risk injury from snow and ice, you also risk hypothermia [low body temperature] if you are exposed to freezing water.

Soccer

Quit While You're Ahead

I still remember the pain and fear in my family's eyes and the panic in my soul. I could hear my heart beat real fast and loud. You didn't need a stethoscope to hear it. I sure learned a lesson that day, and it is still frightening to think about it.

It was a hot summer day, and my family and I were playing a game of soccer. I was tired and couldn't go on anymore, but I forced myself to keep playing. That was my tragic mistake, a mistake that cost me my whole summer—and my arm along with it.

I had the ball and was running. I couldn't see the bumps or cracks in the ground in front of me because the ball was blocking my view, and I was dizzy from all that running. Suddenly I tripped and fell face first into the ground with my arms behind me. When I fell, I heard a loud CRACK! I didn't think of the noise at first, but when I got up I couldn't feel my arm. When I looked at it, I saw it was twisted! I screamed, and everyone rushed over. They thought I had injured a muscle or something because my arm popped back into place. I calmed down and got up, but my arm popped out of place again. I knew it was broken because I had broken it before. I calmly said that my arm was broken and that I had to go to the hospital. I was there within minutes.

The doctors said I had broken both bones. I had a splint and a cast for a month. Because I was growing and the bones wouldn't heal by themselves, the doctors said I needed screws in my arm. They operated to put the screws in, and I had a cast on again for another month.

I learned never to play sports in areas where the ground is bumpy or has roots sticking up. Also, I learned that I should stop playing when I am tired. When your body can't go anymore, don't force yourself, because your body knows when to stop. I sure learned a lesson. I hope you learned one, too, from my story.

Ronald Pastor, 13
Stratford

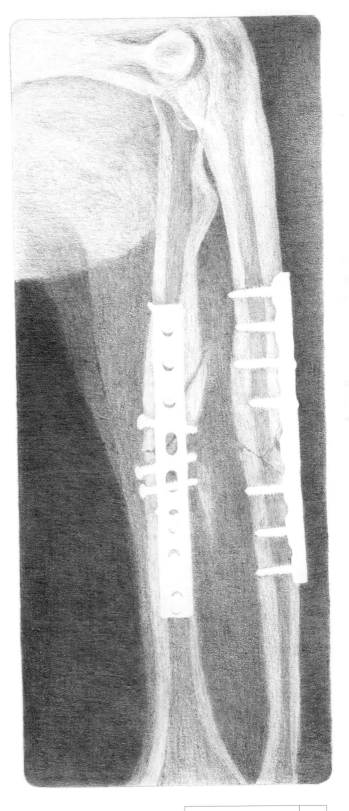

Streets + Parking Lots

Close Call

Just imagine that you're talking on the phone with your best friend, when, all of a sudden, you hear horrible screams—the screams of your twelve-, seven-, and five-year-old cousins. At first, I thought they were playing, but after the second scream, I knew something was wrong. I hung up the phone immediately and raced out the door. They were all crying, then yelling my name. I started to cry, my body shook, and I couldn't see straight. Rosanne, my twelve-year-old cousin, yelled, "Grandma!" My cousin Taylor yelled, "Mom, stop!" My five-year-old cousin yelled, "Oh, my God!"

My cousin Timmy, who was only three, was laying on the ground, his arm covered with blood, crying as my mother ran toward us. My aunt shot out of the car, screaming, and picked up Timmy. My mother took Timmy from her, and my aunt ran into my grandmother's arms. We held her and Timmy close and told them that everything would be fine. All my aunt kept saying was that she almost killed him, that she almost killed her baby. She really didn't, though. After the ambulance came, they took Timmy to the hospital. All he came out with was a bandaged arm, because all the skin was scaped off. Thank God.

When this horrible event took place, it was raining, and my aunt told my cousins to stay in my grandmother's kitchen while she backed the car into the garage. But Timmy didn't listen. He ran out of the house because he forgot his toy outside. He ran toward the car while my aunt was backing up and ran into the back of the car. The impact of bumping into the car threw him onto the ground.

My advice to the world is, stay away from cars when they are backing up. Just because you see them, you shouldn't assume the driver can see you. And listen to your parents when they tell you to say put. You can always buy a new toy, but you can never replace a person.

Jessica Hurlburt, 14
Pawcatuck

Dr. Baker's Comment:

Injuries from automobiles are the most common causes of death in children. Jessica has offered some good advice about how to prevent them. First, never walk or run in back or in front of a car while the engine is running. As Jessica tells us, you should never assume that the driver is able to see you. Second, when you are instructed to do something by an adult, be sure to do it. Many injuries—like Timmy's— could have been avoided if children had followed the advice of those who knew better.

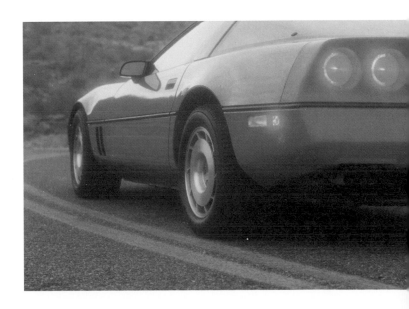

Both Ways

One day this summer, my family and I went out for breakfast at my favorite restaurant. When we were done, my mom took my sister outside to look at the water fountain. I ran back to the table to pay the tip with Daddy. Then, I ran outside to catch up with my mom and sister. They were across the parking lot. I ran right between some cars and smacked my nose on a car that was driving by.

I remember lying on the ground. Lots of people started screaming, and a woman came up to me and said I shouldn't move. I saw Mommy and Daddy crying, and then some police cars and an ambulance came. I had to lie there a long time. They put this Styrofoam thing around my neck. I remember that I didn't cry. I just kept lying there, feeling sad. They put me on a stretcher and carried me to the ambulance. The driver said it would be like a hayride and I shouldn't be scared. The ride to the hospital was bumpy, and I had to keep my nose scrunched up because of the thing around my neck and the blood dripping down.

When we got to the hospital, some people checked me out and told me I was really lucky. When we got home, Mommy made me write a letter to the man driving the car to tell him I was okay and that I was sorry I forgot to look both ways. The police visited me a few days later and gave me a safety bear so I could remember how to act safe. So please, look both ways—and always stay with your parents in a parking lot!

Brenna Marie Marcoux, 6
Glastonbury

Dr. Baker's Comment:

Fortunately, Brenna was not seriously injured, although she could have been. Sometimes, it is difficult to be patient and careful, but the extra time it takes is well worth it. Always look both ways before entering any street or parking lot. Don't ever walk into an area with traffic if you cannot see clearly—in both directions!

Then

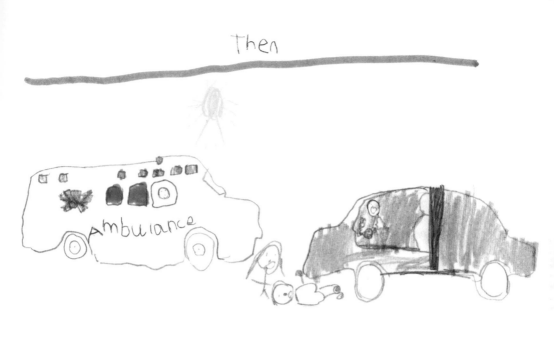

Ambulance

Now

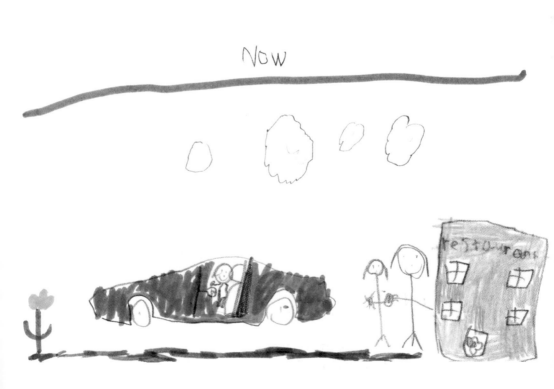

restaurant

Swimming

The Day I Almost Drowned

One day, about two years ago, I was walking across a stream with a friend. It thought it was a very shallow stream, until I put my foot in the water and fell in. My friend thought I was just kidding, so he watched and laughed.

While I was under the water trying to get out, there was a current pulling me farther down. It was so dark that I couldn't even find a rock to pull myself up. At last, I finally grabbed hold of a rock and pulled myself up—but the current was so strong that it pulled me right back under. I was so scared. I was losing all my breath. Then, my hand hit another rock, and I pulled myself out. I was crying and shaking.

What I think could have prevented this is if I had not gone into the stream in the first place. Second, I should have been with an adult at that time. So be careful, and stay close to an adult when you are near water!

Kara Greenwood, 12
Trumbull

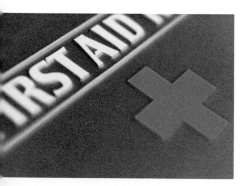

Just in Time

My story is about a thirteen-year-old boy that I didn't even know. He was swimming by himself at a public pool. I know that no one was with him, and his parents weren't home. Someone told me later that he didn't know how to swim. It was a day that neither he nor I will ever forget.

I had just gotten out of school, and my friend Alicia was with me. I love to swim, and we were at the pool for less than a minute when I jumped in. I saw an object at the bottom of the pool. At first, I thought it was a towel or a shirt, but then I realized it wasn't. I noticed that someone else was also staring at the bottom of the pool, so I thought I'd check it out.

When I got closer, I realized that it was a boy! I grabbed him the way my dad's girlfriend had shown me the day before. I brought him to the surface. I yelled to Alicia to get help. The pool attendant and a woman at the pool helped resuscitate [revive] him until the ambulance arrived. The next day, I went to the hospital to see him. He was fine, and his parents couldn't stop saying thank-you.

I received a reward from the mayor, the State of Connecticut, and my school. I just recently received a reward from the National Legion.

I'm glad that this didn't happen to me or my brother. No one should be so careless as to go anywhere near a pool if they can't swim. My advice is, don't be like that boy. Only swim if you can and always with an adult.

Amanda Rapuano, 13
East Haven

Dr. Smothers's Comment:
What a scare for that boy and his family! Thanks to Amanda, fortunately, he survived. Too many children drown each year. Adults that can swim must supervise children around or near a pool, beach, lake, pond, or stream. Be sure to always wear a life vest unless you swim very well.

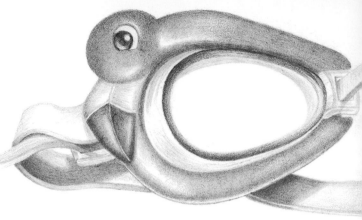

One False Step

One hot, sunny, summer day, my family and I were spending the day at the pool. I was two years old and wore a life vest. I hated my life vest. It was the ugliest orange you could imagine, and it stuck to my skin. Whenever I took it off, it would sting just like ripping tape off my skin.

I was floating around the pool with my dad. I was trying to do tricks like handstands or flips for my mom. When I became tired of that, I got out of the pool. I remember my mom saying, "If you are staying out for now, you can take off your life vest." So I did.

A while later, I was walking by the edge of the pool. I got too close to the edge, and before I knew it, I fell in. Because I wasn't wearing my life vest, I sank to the bottom. I was drowning. I was so little I made no splashing noise at all when I fell in. I was scared!

My older brother noticed me and yelled for my parents as he jumped into the pool after me. The next thing I remember was my dad pulling me up, while my mom was yelling, "Are you all right?" I was crying but okay. Now I know better—always be careful when you are near a pool.

Stephanie Rogowski, 11
Shelton

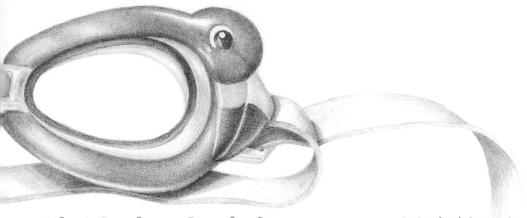

What Good are Goggles?

This is a true story about my friend Jillie. She was swimming (without any goggles) and swam into the side of the pool. After she hit her head, she became unconscious and stopped breathing.

Luckily, her brother saw the accident and called their mom. The first thing her mom did was call 911. Then she pulled Jillie out of the pool. Soon, the ambulance and the paramedics came. They gave Jillie mouth-to-mouth resuscitation, put her in the ambulance, and drove her to the hospital.

The doctors put Jillie on a ventilator. Because Jillie couldn't breathe by herself, the ventilator had to breathe for her. She spent three days in the hospital, resting and getting stronger. When Jillie was able to breathe on her own, her parents took her home. Since then, she has been perfectly fine.

I learned two things from Jillie's experience. First, always make sure that there is an adult with you when you are swimming. If Jillie's mom hadn't been there to pull her out, she would have drowned. Second, if you can't open your eyes or see clearly underwater, wear goggles. If you learn these lessons, you will be able to have fun *and* stay safe while you are swimming.

Olivia Schweitzer, 9
Woodbridge

Dr. Smothers's Comment:
Pools can be a lot of fun, but they can also be dangerous places. Kids should always wear goggles or swim with their eyes open. In case of an emergency, be sure you call 911 right away, as Jillie's mom did. These simple lessons can save lives.

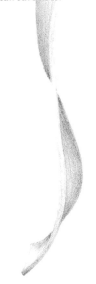

Trampolines

Dr. Smothers's Comment:

Nicole and Amy point out many of the dangers of trampolines. I agree that they can be fun, but in the emergency room, we see many injuries caused by playing on trampolines, and some are very serious.

The safest thing is to not play on trampolines at all. But if you do, as Nicole says, never have more than one person on the trampoline at a time, don't try dangerous flips, and always have adult supervision. You should also wear a helmet, wrist guards, and knee and elbow pads.

Boiiing!

The Saturday before Thanksgiving, I was at my cousins' house. My two cousins, Justin, age 13, and David, age 10, had three friends sleep over the night before. We were all outside in the backyard jumping on the trampoline. My uncle was inside watching television. Everything was going peacefully, until Justin fell off the trampoline, head first. I tried to stop him by grabbing his legs, but he kicked his legs suddenly, and I was flung off, too. I heard my arm crack and I started to scream and cry. My uncle came rushing out with the phone and called 911. Paramedics came within 15 minutes and took me to the hospital.

I got two shots and some X rays. The X rays were the most painful because the doctors kept moving my arm. Later, I was taken to a small room where the nicest doctor put my arm in a plaster cast. The cast was on for about 12 weeks.

My advice to kids is all the basic stuff you should already know—such as calling 911 and staying calm in an emergency. Using your common sense is a big thing. You should know better than to have five people on a trampoline at one time. Make sure someone is always spotting you. If no one can spot you, then go do something else. Think before you act. You can get hurt.

Nicole Miller, 12
Burlington

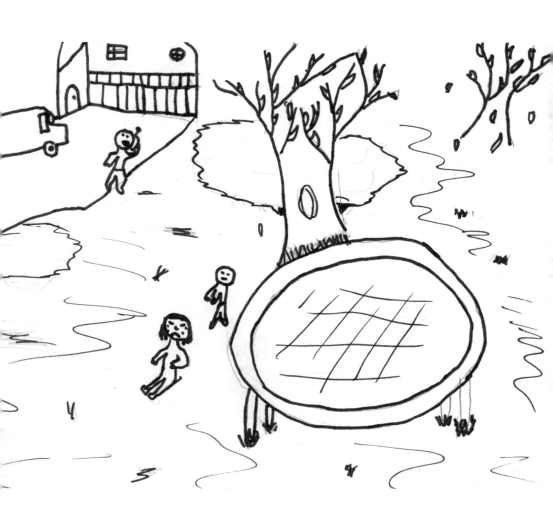

Jumping with Joe and Ninja

One morning, I was jumping on my trampoline in my backyard with my brother. He had his action figures on it, too. They were bouncing up and down while we were jumping. I decided to do a flip, but was trying to avoid the G. I. Joe in front of me and the Ninja Turtle behind me, so I moved over to the right while I was still in the air. I thought I would land on the trampoline, but instead my body slammed fiercely onto the ground. I stayed on the ground, not able to move, yelling for my mother. She ran outside to help me into the house.

I lay down on the couch while my mom looked at my collarbone, which I had landed on. She guessed that I had broken it. She helped me to the car and took me to Med-Now. The people there brought me into the X-ray room and took the pictures. The doctors confirmed that my collarbone was broken. The orthopedic surgeon gave me a brace that I had to wear around my shoulders.

Eventually, my collarbone healed fully and was back to normal. To this day, I still have a bump there, but it will be gone by the time I get married.

That accident was very unpleasant. I want to advise you not to do flips on trampolines, and don't jump on one when something else is on it that could cause an accident.

Amy Warren, 13
Stratford

Runaway Baby

One day, my brother, who was eleven months old, was inside the house in his walker. My dad went out to the backyard and shut the screen door behind him. My mom was in the house with my brother and me. She was doing something and didn't see my brother open the screen door. He went out onto the deck and toward the stairs. The walker rolled down the stairs, and my brother hit his face on the ground. My mom took him to the emergency room, and my dad stayed home with me.

At the hospital, they checked to make sure my brother didn't break his nose. He didn't break anything, but his face was bruised. They gave my mom ointment to put on his face.

My mom and dad made sure something like this would never happen again by putting another lock on the door. When there are young children around, you have to be extra careful that there is nothing they can get into and get hurt. Put extra locks on doors and also locks on cabinets. You could also put gates across any doorways near stairs.

Stephanie Rogers, 14
East Haven

Dr. Kennedy's Comment:

On first thought, infant walkers are great. They allow the little ones to zoom around the house and get to places that they wouldn't be able to get to until they became toddlers. But the story of Stephanie's brother—and the stories of thousands of other children like him— make us think again.

Pediatricians would like to see infant walkers become extinct—not because they are not fun, but because of all the injuries they cause. Thanks for your message, Stephanie. It helps all of us doctors in our "war against walkers."

Tips for Safety

from the staff of
Yale New Haven Health

Basic Safety

1. Wear a helmet when you ride a bicycle or go skating or sledding—and never ride double with anyone.
2. Don't play with guns. If someone in your home has a gun, make sure it is locked away—unloaded.
3. Always wear a seatbelt in a car. Never ride in the car when the driver has been drinking alcohol. Never drive a car if you have been drinking alcohol.
4. Don't eat or drink anything that doesn't have a label you can read and understand. Don't take medicine that belongs to someone else. Make sure you know the phone number for the nearest Poison Center.
5. Look both ways before crossing the street. Cross only at intersections.
6. Don't swim alone. Be careful where you dive. Wear goggles.
7. Wear the right kind of safety equipment to play sports.
8. Don't play with matches, stoves, or firecrackers. Make sure there are working smoke detectors, carbon-monoxide detectors, and fire extinguishers in your home. Have a family escape plan in case there is a fire in your home. If there are young children in your home, make sure there are no matches or lighters within their reach.
9. Be careful when you play outside. Don't climb on fences, ladders, or trees. And don't jump from playground equipment.
10. Use tools or machines only with adult supervision.

Bicycle Safety

1. Always wear a helmet.
2. Look both ways before you start riding and after you stop.
3. Ride in a straight line.
4. Don't swerve.
5. Concentrate.
6. Ride with traffic.
7. Stop at stop signs.
8. Warn pedestrians that you are riding.
9. Brake and slow down before you turn.
10. Signal before turning.
11. Don't ride with anyone on the handlebars.
12. Listen for sounds.
13. Check out the bicycle before you ride. Make sure the brakes work and the tires are inflated properly.
14. Be sure you have the right shoes on—no sandals or bare feet.
15. Tuck in or roll up long pants so they won't get caught in the chain or wheels.
16. Keep loose strings or straps away from the wheels and chain.
17. When you get to an intersection, walk your bicycle across the street.

Car Safety

1. Always wear a seatbelt.
2. Don't ride with someone who has been drinking alcohol.
3. Don't drive if you have been drinking alcohol.
4. Don't stick your head, hands, or feet out of the windows of a moving car.
5. Look before you close the car door—and don't open doors before the car has stopped completely.

Sports Safety

1. Always wear the proper equipment when playing sports.
2. Warm up before you play.
3. Be alert during practice, warm-ups, and games.
4. Know where the boundaries of the field are, especially walls or fences. Play in safe, level, open areas.

Tips for Baby-sitters

1. Always be prepared for an emergency.
2. Be sure you have a phone number to reach the child's parents. Call for help if you have questions or a problem.
3. Don't open the door to strangers.
4. Never leave a child alone.
5. Don't give a child medicine or food unless parents say it is okay.

Water Safety

1. Learn how to swim.
2. Don't swim alone. Make sure a lifeguard or another adult is watching.
3. Be careful where you dive. Jumping in is safer.
4. Always wear a life jacket when you are in a boat.
5. Be careful when you play near the ocean. Only swim in areas marked for swimming and only when a lifeguard is on duty.
6. Wear goggles or swim with your eyes open.

In Case of Emergency

1. Always stay calm.
2. Think about what you are doing.
3. If there is a fire, get out of the house and call for help.
4. When you call 911 for help, stay on the phone until the operator tells you to hang up.
5. If you are on fire, stop what you are doing, drop to the ground and roll. (STOP, DROP AND ROLL.)
6. If someone is not moving, talk to them. If they don't talk back, touch them and talk to them. If they still don't talk, call for help.

Help and Information

Emergency	911
Poison Control	(in CT) 800-343-2722

Your Doctor

_____

Your Dentist

_____

Neighbors, Baby-sitters, and other Adults

_____

_____

Physician Referral Lines

Bridgeport Hospital	203-384-444
	or toll free 888-357-2396
Greenwich Hospital	203-863-DOCS
Yale-New Haven Children's Hospital	203-688-2000
	or toll free 888-700-6543
Web address	www.ynhh.org/ynhhs/ynhhs.html

Credits

Published by Yale New Haven Health

Editors
  Douglas Baker, M.D.
  Thomas Kennedy, M.D.
  Kevin Smothers, M.D.

Associate Editors
  Kenneth Best
  Deborah Cannarella

Cover and Book Design
  Jeanne Criscola/Criscola Design

Cover Illustration
  Richie Hales Urtz

Illustrations
  Richie Hales Urtz
  pp. 10, 14, 21, 24-25, 28-29, 38, 40-41, 47, 53, 55, 62-63, 67, 69, 71,
  76-77, 83, 84, 88-89, 92, 95, 102-103

Illustrations by Authors
  Beth Maco, pp. 5, 60
  Melissa Harrigan, pp. 6, 26
  Brittany Hallenbeck, p. 13
  Isaac Civitello, p. 18
  Jeremy Godenzi, p. 35
  Timothy Stobierski, p. 37
  Jason Cote, p. 43
  Hillary Ganoe, p. 50
  Dave Kramer, p. 59
  Rebekah Prenoveau, p. 87
  Brenna Marie Marcoux, p. 99
  Nicole Miller, p. 105

Printing
  Harty Press

Set in TheMix and TheSerif.
Printed on Garda Silk.

Visit the Web site for Yale New Haven Health
www.ynhh.org/ynhhs/ynhhs.html